DO YOU KNOW WHAT TO EAT?

*To Nissa Beth, who shares her enthusiasm for and knowledge about tasty,
nutritious food with her family and friends.*

Published in 2016 by Enslow Publishing, LLC
101 W. 23rd Street, Suite 240, New York, NY 10011

Copyright © 2016 by Kathlyn Gay

All rights reserved.

No part of this book may be reproduced by any means without the written permission of the publisher.

Library of Congress Cataloging-in-Publication Data
Gay, Kathlyn.
 Do you know what to eat? / Kathlyn Gay.
  pages cm. — (Got issues?)
 Audience: 12-up.
 Audience: Grade 7 to 8.
 Includes bibliographical references and index.
 Summary: "Discusses the difficulties facing those with eating problems and includes the history of,
symptoms, treatments, nutrition, and ways to help"—Provided by publisher.
 ISBN 978-0-7660-6987-9
 1. Nutrition—United States—Juvenile literature. 2. Obesity—United States—Juvenile literature. 3. Food
habits—United States—History—Juvenile literature. I. Title.
 RA645.O23G39 2016
 613.2—dc23
                                   2015011773

Printed in the United States of America

To Our Readers: We have done our best to make sure all Web site addresses in this book were active and
appropriate when we went to press. However, the author and the publisher have no control over and assume
no liability for the material available on those Web sites or on any Web sites they may link to. Any comments
or suggestions can be sent by e-mail to customerservice@enslow.com.

Portions of this book originally appeared in the book *The Scoop on What to Eat: What You Should Know
About Diet and Nutrition.*

Disclaimer: For many of the images in this book, the people photographed are models. The depictions do
not imply actual situations or events.

Photo Credits: 2xSamara.com/Shutterstock.com, p. 27; alexpro9500/Shutterstock.com, p. 25; Anna
Omelchenko/Shutterstock.com, p. 87; bogdan ionescu/Shutterstock.com, p. 13; ChooseMyPlate.gov,
p. 53; Elena Elisseeva/Shutterstock.com, p. 75; fotoknips/Shutterstock.com, p. 72; Guy Shapira/
Shutterstock.com, p. 56; Iakov Filimonov/Shutterstock.com, p.90; Jack Chabraszewski/Shutterstock.com,
p. 85; Jason Stitt/Shutterstock.com, p. 3; Kekyalyayen/Shutterstock.com, p. 35; Krzycho/Shutterstock.
com, p. 51; Maya Kruchankova/Shutterstock.com, p. 35; Monkey Business Images/Shutterstock.com,
pp. 7, 59, 80; MSPhotographic/Shutterstock.com, p. 32; National Center for Chronic Disease Prevention
and Health Promotion, p. 10; nenetus/Shutterstock.com, p. 62; Nomad_Soul/Shutterstock.com, p. 18;
PathDoc/Shutterstock.com, p. 41; Robert Kneschke/Shutterstock.com, p. 69; Umkeher/Shutterstock, p.
90; violeta pasat/Shutterstock.com, p. 78; VTT Studio/Shutterstock.com, p. 42; Zurijeta/Shutterstock.
com, p. 35.

Cover Credit: Jason Stitt/Shutterstock.com (African-American girl holding apple and burger).

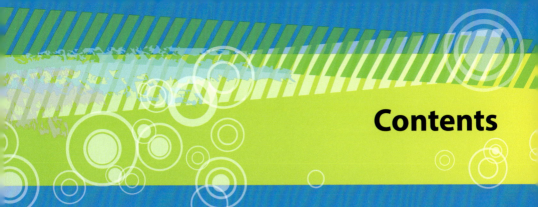

Contents

Chapter 1 Eating While Socializing 7

Chapter 2 What's in a Name? 13

Chapter 3 Our Eating Practices 27

Chapter 4 Poor Eating Habits Impair Health 35

Chapter 5 Dangerous Eating Behaviors 42

Chapter 6 Do You Eat for Good Health? 51

Chapter 7 Dieting Dos and Don'ts 62

Chapter 8 What Vegetarians Eat 72

Chapter 9 Getting Enough Exercise 80

Chapter 10 Enjoy a Healthy Lifestyle 87

Chapter Notes 94
Glossary 103
For More Information............105
Further Reading 108
Index 109

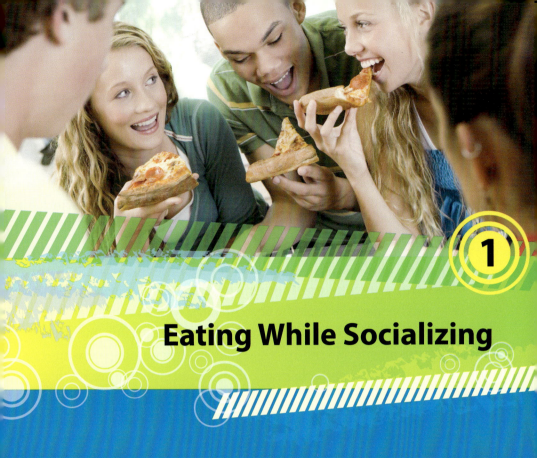

Eating While Socializing

In most areas of the United States, food is part of social and sports events, as well as at family gatherings and national celebrations. In fact, whenever and wherever people gather, food and beverages are likely to be consumed.

For example, if you are a sports fan—whether it is football, baseball, hockey, or basketball—one part of enjoying the game as a spectator usually means hailing a vendor for refreshments. If you are with friends or family, you are likely to share purchases, such as chips or popcorn.

If you like video games, you and your friends may gather to compete and indulge in snacks and drinks.

If you go to a movie at a theater with friends or family, you might snack on a large tub or bucket of popcorn.

Do You Know What to Eat?

If you take part in or attend a school graduation, you may go to a congratulatory dinner, a picnic for graduates, or another food-based event.

If you like to meet with classmates or friends after the school day is over, you may join your group at a favorite pizza or other fast food place.

If you are invited to a birthday party, you, like most guests, will probably expect part of the festivities to include cake, ice cream, and a soft drink.

In short, food is part of many occasions because it helps people interact and share with one another. However, the old saying "Eat, drink, and be merry" should be accompanied with a bit of caution. Numerous experts on food and nutrition say have fun, but be aware that some foods and beverages do little or nothing for your health and could even be harmful. For example, people are often tempted to eat and drink more than they need or really want when they socialize. If people overeat too often, they may gain unwanted pounds. Or if someone is a diabetic or has an allergy, she or he might eat foods that could cause harmful reactions.

Besides the social issue, it is common for many Americans to eat more than usual when they are stressed or unhappy. Other behavioral, economic, and cultural factors related to food may also lead to diverse health problems.

Overweight Americans

For at least three decades, health experts in the United States have raised concerns about the increasing number of Americans who are overweight or obese. Studies show that Americans are fatter than most other populations worldwide. To be considered overweight, people must have a body weight that exceeds standards set for a certain group. In other words, their weight is greater than what is generally considered a healthy range, which determined by their age and height. Sometimes athletes or bodybuilders can be overweight because of excess muscle, but they are not obese. According to a

Eating While Socializing

report on childhood obesity in the United States in 2011 to 2012 by the US Centers for Disease Control and Prevention (CDC), "Childhood obesity prevalence remains high. Overall, obesity among our nation's young people, aged 2 to 19 years, has not changed significantly since 2003-2004 and remains at about 17 percent." [1]

In some cases, a physician may diagnose a person as having a medical condition known as morbid obesity. This means the person is severely obese—one hundred pounds or more over the ideal body weight. Such a person is at great risk of obesity-related health conditions or serious diseases.

How to Calculate BMI

The most commonly used method to calculate if a person is overweight or obese is the body mass index (BMI). Adults may use a table showing height in inches along a vertical column and weight in pounds across a horizontal column. The BMI is indicated at the top of the table.

However, standard BMI tables for children and teenagers are different from those used by adults because as children grow their proportion of fat weight changes. It may be high at age eleven but lower at age thirteen as they grow taller. Thus when determining BMI for children and teenagers, health care professionals may use what are frequently called BMI-for-age charts.

Curved lines on a chart show percentiles, or values on a scale of 100. A person's BMI plotted on the chart indicates whether her or his BMI exceeds or equals others of the same age and gender. If a ten-year-old girl is in the 50th percentile, this means that 50 percent of girls of the same age have a lower BMI. A sixteen-year-old boy might be in the 60th percentile, so 60 percent of boys of the same age have a lower BMI. Both female and male young people are considered overweight if their BMI is in the 95th percentile or higher.

The increasing BMI rates of Americans have raised health concerns. Being overweight or obese boosts the risk of having many diseases and adverse health conditions, including but not limited to

Do You Know What to Eat?

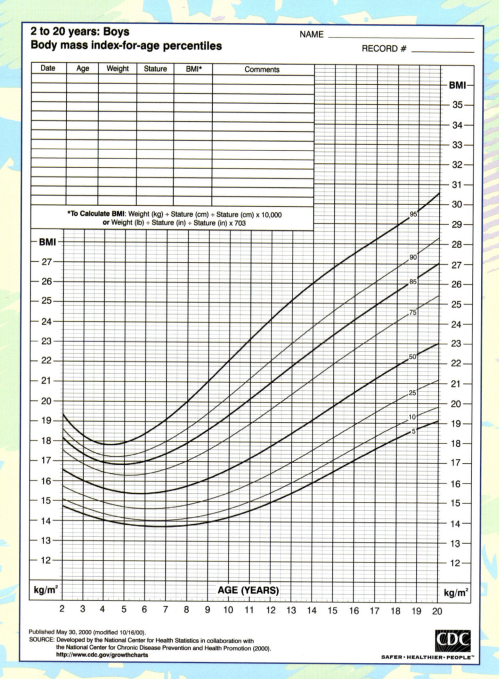

The Body Mass Index (BMI) uses the factors of height and weight to determine whether a person is at a healthy weight. For teens, the BMI is compared against others in the same age group and gender.

diabetes, heart disease, stroke, arthritis, and some cancers. Severe obesity can also cause breathing problems because the lungs decrease in size. Mowing the lawn, raking, climbing stairs, and exercising become difficult. As one TV commercial shows, it is like an elephant sitting on your chest.

Other Health Concerns

Many teenagers face eating disorders—destructive behaviors to lose weight that can lead to serious illnesses and sometimes even death. In addition, fad diets and controversial detox diet plans designed to rid the body of toxic materials may impact one's health in an adverse way no matter what advertisements say about the benefits.

Questions also arise about eating out or buying carryout foods; are these practices good for a person's health? And who has not heard about junk food and fast food—are they the same thing and are they unhealthy? Are packaged convenience meals healthy?

Whatever types of meals people eat, it is important to consume nutritious food that provides the vitamins, minerals, protein, and other nutrients the body needs. New York City's Department of Health and Mental Hygiene has a website called Teen Speak where teenagers express their opinions on that topic. Carlos, a sixteen-year-old says, "If I eat junk food, my body feels heavy and I have no energy. I found that eating good food can really help me feel energized." Petry, age fifteen, says, "People forget about having 5 servings of fruits or vegetables every day to get the vitamins and minerals that are essential for a healthy body." Seventeen-year-old Shayanne says, "I stopped eating junk food and started eating Mom's healthier cooking. Now, I'm strong and fit and I'm looking like a model." [2]

The Upside of Healthy Eating

Besides the helpful comments above, chapters in this book cover other positive approaches to healthy eating. For example, some teens and adults—admittedly a minority—follow a vegetarian or

Do You Know What to Eat?

semi-vegetarian regimen and consider it not only healthy but also enjoyable.

Maybe you are hesitant to try healthy foods because the word healthy makes you think of broccoli, brussels sprouts, spinach, or other vegetables with a reputation for being good for you but not particularly tasty. Well, think again. There are delicious and healthy items, such as fruit smoothies, breakfast burritos made with whole-wheat tortillas, baked corn chips with mango salsa or black bean dip, veggie pizza, and apple slices with peanut butter and raisins. Numerous healthy choices are increasingly available in grocery stores, vending machines, and school cafeterias.

Finally, to be in top form, there are suggestions included in this book for a nutritious, healthy eating plan. But first it is important to know what kind of foods do little to improve health and what kinds provide the nutrients your body needs to function properly.

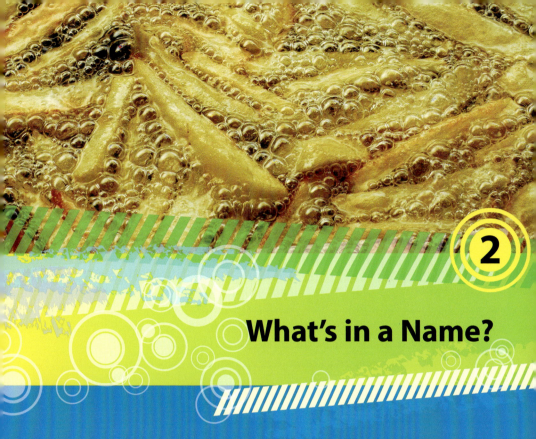

2

What's in a Name?

You've no doubt seen the terms junk food and fast food. Numerous books, articles, and films have described these foods. But what are they and what do the terms mean?

One definition of junk food is any food or beverage that provides excess calories, fat, and salt and has little nutrient value. These foods include snacks such as high-fat potato chips, many fried foods, and candy bars. Sugary beverages are in the junk food category, as well. They do not contain fat but are high in empty calories—calories that do not provide any nutrients. These foods can be found in supermarkets, convenience stores, fast food restaurants, and school vending machines, although some schools are eliminating junk foods. Nevertheless, small portions of these snacks every now and then are not detrimental if the rest of your daily diet is nutritious and healthy. Plus, you exercise to keep your weight in balance.

Do You Know What to Eat?

Is Fast Food Junk Food?

Frequently the term fast food is used to mean junk food, but fast food and junk food are not necessarily the same thing. For example, some fast foods could be healthy choices, such as packaged salads found at restaurants like McDonald's and Wendy's. Another fast food item is pizza, which is not necessarily unhealthy. Nutritionist Elaine Magee, who writes for WebMD, says:

> *"Junk food" generally refers to foods that contribute lots of calories but little nutritional value. Of course, what's considered "junk food" depends on whom you ask. Some might say pizza is junk food, for example. But I personally don't think so, since it contributes real food with nutrients, like cheese and tomato sauce. Add whole wheat or part whole wheat crust, plus veggies as a topping, and I'd say pizza completely exits the junk food category.[1]*

On the other hand, some quick, convenient items, such as french fries or sugary soft drinks in fast food restaurants, could be categorized as junk food. While it is seldom easy to order healthy meals at a fast food restaurant, the National Heart, Lung, and Blood Institute (NHLBI) has published a handout that compares a high-calorie food to one lower in calories. One example is a double meat cheeseburger at 1,120 calories; a healthier option would be a grilled chicken sandwich without mayonnaise. A substitute for a medium chocolate milkshake at 500 calories could be a carton of low-fat milk at 110 calories. [2]

Although it is tempting to eat high-fat and sugary foods in fast food restaurants, some people try to choose healthy items. One such person is teenager Astrid who posted a message on Teen Speak in November 2014. She wrote:

> *I think that eating healthy is important because it makes me feel great and it has a long-lasting effect on my body. I started eating healthy because I saw my mother doing it, and I could see how much better it made her feel and how energetic she was, and I*

What's in a Name?

wanted that for myself. At first it was hard because there are so many fast food places and lots of stores that only sell candy, chips, etc. I kept telling myself that I wanted to look and feel better, so I ignored all the fast food places and started eating healthier foods and doing my 30 minutes of walking every day. Now I feel and look better than ever before! [3]

Although fast food restaurants offer plenty of items with low nutritional value, some chains, such as McDonald's, Subway, Taco Bell, Wendy's, and KFC, also offer foods low in sugar, fat, and calories. In fact, federal law requires that these restaurants and others show on their menus the amount of calories in their foods. On November 25, 2014, the US Food and Drug Administration, an agency within the US Department of Health and Human Services, announced in a news release that it had finalized two rules requiring calorie information on menus and menu boards in chain restaurants, similar retail food businesses, and vending machines with twenty or more locations. The rules are required by the 2010 Patient Protection and Affordable Care Act.

"Americans eat and drink about one third of their calories away from home, and people today expect clear information about the products they consume," said FDA Commissioner Margaret A. Hamburg, M.D. "Making calorie information available on chain restaurant menus and vending machines is an important step for public health that will help consumers make informed choices for themselves and their families." [4]

While fast foods are, for the most part, not the best source of nutrition, they can fit into a healthy diet. The trick is to make smart choices whether eating out, at home, or on the school campus.

How to Make Smart Choices

There is no precise definition for smart food, although for this book the expression refers to foods and beverages that help the body function in a healthy manner. Such foods contain essential nutrients, which are chemical substances that are absolutely necessary for our bodies to function effectively. We have to depend on nutrients in our diet because our bodies are not able to produce many of them or cannot produce them in adequate amounts. Basic nutrients include proteins, carbohydrates, fats and oils, minerals, vitamins, and water. Although it may seem strange to consider water a nutrient, it is a nourishing substance that is vital for life.

Good nutrition helps people stay healthy and can prevent heart diseases, fragile bones, and other chronic problems. To be informed about nutrients, here are some brief explanations.

Proteins

According to the Genetics Home Reference handbook:

> Proteins are large, complex molecules that play many critical roles in the body. They do most of the work in cells and are required for the structure, function, and regulation of the body's tissues and organs. Proteins are made up of hundreds or thousands of smaller units called amino acids, which are attached to one another in long chains. There are 20 different types of amino acids that can be combined to make a protein.[5]

Amino acids come in many shapes and sizes and can make thousands of different proteins, but scientists have determined that twenty-two of them are essential for good health. The body makes thirteen of these amino acids, but the other nine must come from food.

Primarily proteins build and repair body tissues from hair and skin to bones and muscles. They also form antibodies that help fight infections. A protein called hemoglobin carries oxygen in the blood to every part of your body. In short, we need proteins for nearly all of our body's activities.

In the United States, the main source of protein is meat with beef at the top of the list. Pork and poultry are other major protein sources. Dairy foods, fish, and eggs provide protein, as do grains, beans, nuts, and seeds. Along with beans, other vegetables contain some protein, including broccoli, cauliflower, carrots, corn, garlic, and mushrooms.

Carbohydrates

Carbohydrates, or carbs for short, provide most of the energy our bodies need and all of the energy our brains need. Carbohydrates are made up of carbon, oxygen, and hydrogen; they combine to make sugar molecules and come in two types, simple and complex carbohydrates.

Simple carbohydrates consist of one or two sugar molecules while complex carbohydrates are made of long chains of sugar molecules and are usually called starches. The body metabolizes, or breaks down, the sugar molecules in food to produce glucose, or blood sugar, which creates energy for cells, tissues, and organs. Simple carbohydrates, such as those found in fruit and milk, break down quickly and provide a burst of energy. However, the blood glucose can drop quickly also, and a person may feel hungry or tired within a short time. Complex carbohydrates, which are found in foods such as breads and cereals, rice, and legumes (beans, peas, and lentils), break down more slowly and provide energy over a longer period of time.

Fats

Fats are made up of chemical compounds called fatty acids—fats and fatty acids essentially mean the same thing. They have gotten a bad reputation over the past few decades as health experts and food advertisers have warned that too much fat is a health risk. Fatty acids also play a major role in cholesterol levels.

Cholesterol is a soft, waxy substance that our bodies make naturally by manufacturing it in the liver, and it also comes from animal products that we eat, such as meat, fish, and dairy. Plant foods have no cholesterol. Cholesterol is transported in the blood to be used for normal body functions, including the production of hormones and vitamin D.

Cholesterol combines with protein and fatty acids to form high-density lipoproteins (HDL) and low-density lipoproteins (LDL). LDL, often called the bad cholesterol, can stick together to form

Do You Know What to Eat?

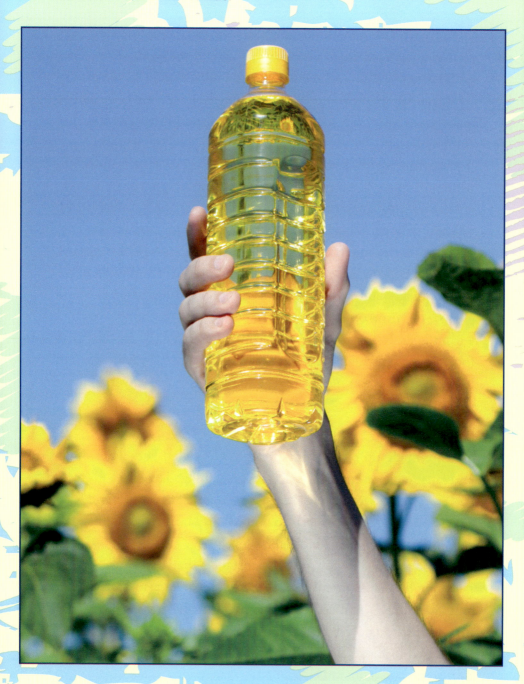

It's not just the items you eat but also how they are cooked that matters for health. Foods cooked in sunflower oil, an unsaturated fat, are healthier than those cooked in butter, a saturated fat.

What's in a Name?

plaque deposits on the walls of a person's blood vessels, which can lead to atherosclerosis, or blocked arteries. HDLs remove used cholesterol from the cells of the body.

Certainly, fats are not all bad. They help the body function properly—they are an energy source (fuel) and are used to produce cell membranes. Fats are also important for healthy hair and skin, provide flavor to foods, help you feel full, and are a source of calories, or energy units in food. Packaged foods and beverages have nutrition fact labels that show the calories per serving and the amount of calories from fat. Serving sizes differ depending on the food or beverage. For example, a serving could be a cup of cereal, a slice of bread, an eight-ounce glass of juice, a tablespoon of mayonnaise, or ten crackers or chips. A label might show that a serving contains 60 calories with 15 of those calories from fat.

According to US dietary guidelines, people should consume no more than 30 percent of their calories from fat based on a daily diet total of 2,000 calories. But labels may not show percentages of fat in various foods. To determine the percentage of calories from fat, divide the number of calories from fat by the total calories and then multiply by 100. Using the total of 60 calories with 15 calories from fat, divide 15 by 60 and multiply by 100. The result is 25 percent of the calories are from fat.

Whatever the percentages, a study by the Harvard School of Public Health found that "the total amount of fat in the diet, whether high or low, isn't really linked with disease. What really matters is the *type of fat* in the diet."[6]

There are four main types of fat or fatty acids, which are chains of carbon atoms with hydrogen atoms attached to them. A saturated fatty acid has the maximum possible number of hydrogen atoms attached to every carbon atom. It is therefore said to be saturated with hydrogen atoms. Saturated fats are solid at room temperature, and they can be found in food from animals, such as lard, butter, cheeses, and other dairy products. They can increase the risk for various diseases, including heart disease. Unsaturated fats—

Do You Know What to Eat?

monounsaturated and polyunsaturated—have fewer hydrogen atoms attached and are found in liquid vegetable oils and fish; they reduce heart disease risks.

Another type of fat is trans fat, which naturally occurs in small amounts in butter, milk products, cheese, and meats. But trans fats are also created artificially by adding hydrogen to vegetable oil.

Check Those Carbs

Calories are not limited to those in fat. They are also found in carbohydrates and protein in food. On the nutrition label, the amounts of nutrients such as fat, carbohydrates, and protein are shown in grams. One gram is about 1/5 of a teaspoon. It takes about five grams to equal a teaspoon.

To determine the total amount of calories in a food serving, check the label again. Near the bottom of most labels is the calorie equivalent for carbohydrates, protein, and fat. There are only 4 calories per gram of protein and 4 calories per gram of carbohydrates while food fat contains 9 calories per gram. The higher amount of calories in fat is one reason for warnings against high-fat food. Suppose the label on a loaf of bread states that one slice (a serving size) has 10 grams of carbohydrates, 2 grams of protein, and one gram of fat. To compute the total calories in the slice of bread, multiply the 10 grams of carbohydrates by 4 calories (per gram), which equals 40 calories. Multiply the 2 grams of protein by 4, and the result is 8 calories. The one gram of fat multiplied by 9 equals 9 calories. To find the total calories add $40 + 8 + 9 = 57$. Thus the 57 calories in one slice of bread are part of the daily total based on a 2,000 calorie diet.

Not everyone needs the same number of calories for good health, however. A teenager playing school sports may need 3,000 to 3,500 calories a day, but a less active person may require fewer than 2,000. When people take in more calories than they burn, they gain weight; they lose weight when they consume fewer calories than they use.

Professor Walter Willet, chair of the Department of Nutrition at the Harvard School of Public Health, briefly explained in *Scientific American* how the artificial process began:

> In 1901 German chemist Wilhelm Normann discovered the process of partial hydrogenation, which converts inexpensive liquid vegetable oils into shortenings and margarines and creates trans fats as a by-product. Because these cheaper, longer-lasting products mimicked the traditional cooking fats of European and North American cuisines, many countries quickly incorporated them into their food supplies. . . . It took decades for scientists to realize how deadly trans fats could be.[7]

Trans fats boost the LDL or bad cholesterol in the blood. Eating trans fats increases the risk of developing heart disease and is "also associated with a higher risk of developing type 2 diabetes," according to the American Heart Association.[8]

For years, the FDA has required food manufacturers to list the amount of trans fat on nutrition labels, and some countries and cities, such as New York, Boston, and Cambridge, have banned trans fats in restaurant meals, some delis, and bakeries. In November 2013, the FDA ruled that partially hydrogenated oils were not safe and should be banned from the nation's food supply, but as of December 2014 the ruling was not yet permanent.

To comply with the FDA ruling, some snack manufacturers have switched to unsaturated fats, such as canola (made from rapeseed), sunflower, soybean, or corn oil. A variety of restaurants serving fried foods have also replaced saturated fats with the unsaturated kind. Many large national chains, such as Kentucky Fried Chicken, McDonald's, Starbucks, and Dunkin' Donuts, have removed trans fat from their products.

Fats essential for body functions include omega-3 fatty acids, also known as polyunsaturated fatty acids. Omega-3s are essential for brain function, as well as for normal growth and development.

Do You Know What to Eat?

Professor Frank Sacks at the Harvard School of Public Health explains:

> We need omega-3 fatty acids for numerous normal body functions, such as controlling blood clotting and building cell membranes in the brain, and since our bodies cannot make omega-3 fats, we must get them through food. Omega-3 fatty acids are also associated with many health benefits, including protection against heart disease and possibly stroke. New studies are identifying potential benefits for a wide range of conditions including cancer, inflammatory bowel disease, and other autoimmune diseases such as lupus and rheumatoid arthritis.[9]

Since the body does not produce these fats, they must be ingested from such foods as fatty fish (salmon, albacore tuna, sardines, and lake trout are examples), flaxseed, walnuts, canola oil, and non-hydrogenated soybean oil. The American Heart Association (AHA) "recommends eating fish (particularly fatty fish) at least two times (two servings) a week. Each serving is 3.5 ounces cooked, or about ¾ cup of flaked fish. Fatty fish like salmon, mackerel, herring, lake trout, sardines, and albacore tuna are high in omega-3 fatty acids.[9]

Yet nearly all fish and shellfish contain mercury, a toxin. For most people this is not a health problem, although young children, pregnant women, and nursing mothers should avoid some types of fish with high levels of mercury, such as shark, albacore tuna, swordfish, and king mackerel. Instead, safer fish with lower levels of mercury include canned light tuna, shrimp, pollack, and catfish.

Vitamins and Minerals

To assure good health, vitamins and minerals are important components in the diet. These are micronutrients, which means they are needed only in small amounts. But those small amounts help the body grow and develop normally and function properly.

For example, calcium is a mineral required for the development of strong bones. The body cannot produce calcium, so it must be absorbed through foods rich in calcium, such as milk, yogurt, and green leafy vegetables. Vitamin D aids in the calcium absorption process. Sometimes called the sunshine vitamin, vitamin D can be made by the body after exposure to the sun. Some fish are good sources of vitamin D, and small amounts can be found in beef liver, cheese, and egg yolks. Foods fortified with added nutrients provide most of the vitamin D in the US diet. Milk is an example. Ready-to-eat breakfast cereals often contain added vitamin D, as do some brands of orange juice, yogurt, and margarine.

Along with vitamin D, other needed vitamins include A, several B vitamins, C, E, and K. Here is a brief list of what these vitamins do and what food sources provide them:

- Vitamin A helps in the formation and maintenance of healthy teeth, bones, and skin; it also promotes good vision. Vitamin A food sources include lean meats, dairy foods, green and yellow vegetables, and fruits with beta carotene, which converts to vitamin A in the body.
- B vitamins are important for metabolism—the processes within the body that create and use energy. Whole grains, lean meats, poultry, fish, and dairy products are some good sources of B vitamins.
- Vitamin C promotes healthy teeth and gums, helps the body absorb iron, and aids in healing wounds. Citrus fruits, tomatoes, and green vegetables are some foods that provide vitamin C.
- Vitamin E assists in the production of red blood cells. Vegetable oils, nuts, seeds, and green vegetables are some foods that contain vitamin E.
- Vitamin K is important as a coagulant—it helps stop bleeding after an injury or a nosebleed. Food sources include cabbage, cauliflower, and leafy green vegetables.

Do You Know What to Eat?

Minerals

Calcium is just one of more than a dozen minerals our bodies need. Others are iodine, iron, magnesium, phosphorus, potassium, selenium, and zinc. These are their functions and food sources:

- Iodine is used by the thyroid gland to produce hormones, and it aids in growth. Fish, shrimp, dairy products, and grains are rich in iodine.
- Iron is essential for the formation of hemoglobin, which carries oxygen to cells, and it helps prevent anemia. Some food sources are red meats, fish, eggs, and leafy green vegetables.
- Magnesium provides numerous metabolic functions and is needed for normal bone growth and a healthy nervous system. Whole grains, leafy green vegetables, nuts, beans, bananas, and apricots are some foods that contain magnesium.
- Phosphorus aids in blood clotting, bone and teeth formation, cell growth, contraction of the heart muscle, normal heart rhythm, and kidney function. It assists the body in the utilization of vitamins and the conversion of food into energy and is involved in virtually all physiological chemical reactions.
- Potassium is an important electrolyte in the blood that is needed for a healthy nervous system and helps regulate blood pressure and the proper functioning of the heart and liver. Most foods contain some potassium, but bananas, oranges, orange juice, and dried fruits are especially good sources.
- Selenium helps fight cell damage and is needed to maintain the immune system. Sources include fish, shellfish, red meat, liver, chicken, and eggs.
- Zinc helps keep the immune system functioning and is needed for cell division, growth, and healing of wounds. Oysters and other seafood, meat, eggs, and whole wheat products are some food sources of zinc.

What's in a Name?

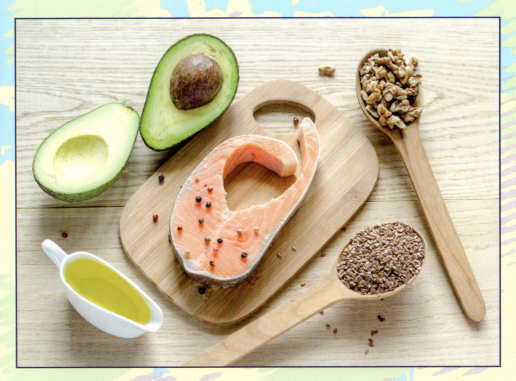

Omega-3 fatty acids are essential to the function of our bodies. Examples of foods that are good sources of omega-3's are canola oil, avocado, salmon, flaxseed, and walnuts.

Water

Water or other liquids in the diet keep us alive. We can survive for weeks without food but only a few days without fluid intake. All of the body's cells and organs depend on water to function. Water helps to transport foods through the intestinal tract and to eliminate waste. It is a lubricant that helps protect joints, and it regulates body temperature.

Our bodies do not store excess water, so our daily diet should include enough water to maintain good health. A common question is how much water does a person need? The usual answer has been at least eight glasses of water daily. But in recent years, health experts say a variety of beverages help supply the fluids the body needs.

Do You Know What to Eat?

Most fluids come from water, milk, juice, soup, coffee, tea, and other beverages. About 20 percent of water comes from the food we eat, especially fruits and vegetables.

In addition, water needs depend on a person's age, physical activity, and exposure to heat. For example, people can lose water through perspiration during strenuous physical activity in hot weather and would need to increase their daily fluid intake. For most people, thirst is the guide that determines whether to drink water or another beverage.

Educate Yourself

Clearly, making smart choices with foods and beverages involves some knowledge about nutrients, which, as described earlier, can be complex and sometimes difficult to determine. But the work may be done for you under certain circumstances—healthy snacks and drinks are increasingly replacing junk food in vending machines, and restaurant menus are highlighting healthy items. In the school cafeteria, nutritious meals and beverages are offered, although some students opt for school snack bar foods, such as high-fat hot dogs and sugary sodas. For meals prepared at home, fresh and packaged food choices can be based on the US Department of Agriculture's (USDA) MyPlate, which replaced MyPyramid in 2011. Guidelines or plans established by medical organizations, such as the Mayo Clinic, the National Institutes of Health, and WebMD, or by nutritionists and dietitians also help with healthy meal preparation.

There are many campaigns underway to educate Americans about smart foods and beverages that can improve health. It is also important to know why and how we eat in order to avoid situations that prompt us to overindulge, gain weight, and consume unhealthy foods.

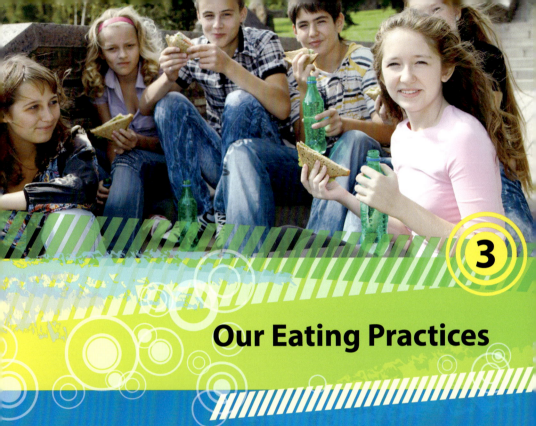

Our Eating Practices

There is no doubt that food is fundamental to our survival. But we have many different ways of consuming food and diverse eating habits. In the United States, our ethnic backgrounds and cultures also influence what, how, and when we eat.

In addition, there are emotional and social reasons we consume certain foods and beverages. Sometimes people eat to relieve stress or to calm emotions. Other times we eat simply because people around us are doing so. Suppose you had a hearty breakfast, but someone among your family or friends has a box of fresh donuts and invites you to indulge. You are not hungry, but you eat a donut (or maybe two or three) anyway. Being around food—seeing and smelling it—can prompt a person to eat even though she or he feels full.

Food is also an important part of our social lives. Our eating behaviors often are related to our social networks—our friends,

Do You Know What to Eat?

classmates, relatives, and others with whom we associate on a regular basis.

"Sharing food is instrumental in creating social groups, and it forms loyalties and obligations that are so intimately tied to our being that we often overlook the power of food to maintain and create those relationships," writes Gillian Crowther in her 2013 book *Eating Culture: An Anthropological Guide to Food.* She adds: "There are many styles and contexts of eating that humans enjoy or just employ; at home, with family and friends, or in public with friends and strangers." [1]

These social relationships may have an impact on whether a person eats too much and gains weight. Many people say that when they hang out with friends, they do what everyone else does. Suppose everyone in your group orders pizza; you may go along and do the same or share with others. If all your friends eat salads, perhaps you will make that choice. In other words, most of us are likely to be interacting with our companions rather than paying attention to what we are eating.

Do Friends and Family Make Us Gain Weight?

The Miriam Hospital Weight Control and Diabetes Research Center in Providence, Rhode Island, conducted a study of young adults and found that "overweight and obese young adults between the ages of 18 and 25 were more likely to have overweight romantic partners and best friends and also had more overweight casual friends and family members compared to normal weight peers," sciencedaily. com reported in 2011. "The study also showed [that] overweight and obese young adults who had more social contacts trying to lose weight were more likely to want to lose weight themselves. Social norms for weight loss, such as encouragement and approval from social contacts, account for this association, researchers say." [2]

In earlier studies, researchers from Harvard Medical School and the University of California, San Diego, collected data on more than twelve thousand people over a period of thirty-two years or more.

Our Eating Practices

The scientists concluded that social ties "have a marked influence on weight gain." One of the principal investigators, Nicholas Christakis, a physician and professor of medical sociology at Harvard Medical School, pointed out:

> *Most likely, the interpersonal, social network effects we observe arise not because friends and siblings adopt each other's lifestyles. It's more subtle than that. What appears to be happening is that a person becoming obese most likely causes a change of norms about what counts as an appropriate body size. People come to think that it is okay to be bigger since those around them are bigger, and this sensibility spreads.*

The researchers stressed that their findings were not meant to encourage people to avoid fat friends or to blame someone else for their weight gain. But they did suggest that having a social network of thin people could influence one's eating behavior.[3]

Kelly Brownell disagrees with the Harvard investigators' conclusions. He told a *New York Times* reporter, "I think there's a great risk here in blaming obese people . . . for things that are caused by a terrible environment."[4] In his book *Food Fight*, Brownell describes that environment as "toxic." That is, conditions in the United States and other industrialized countries are conducive to overeating, gaining weight, and putting people at risk for numerous health problems.

One part of that toxic environment is the supersize trend—fast food meals, sandwiches, fries, and superlarge soft drinks, such as the Big Gulp. In 2012, New York City's then-Mayor Michael Bloomberg banned sugary drinks in containers sixteen ounces or larger. But in 2013, the New York Supreme Court ruled that Bloomberg had overstepped his authority and that the ban was unconstitutional because it exempted some businesses and various drinks—milkshakes, for example. Many other items, such as sandwiches and meal portions in restaurants, have increased in size over the past few decades and were not included in the ban.

Do You Know What to Eat?

Another factor in the toxic environment is the widespread publicity given food-eating contests that exploit overeating by contestants who stuff themselves with hot dogs or gorge on pies or other foods just to see who can consume the most. One more factor is the availability of food—often junk food—around the clock in a variety of places, such as twenty-four-hour groceries, gas stations, interstate cafes, drugstores, and even hospital waiting rooms. In addition, the popularity of TV shows, video games, computer chat rooms, and other sedentary activities discourage regular exercise.

Food for Your Mood

In some cases, emotions trigger eating. Have you ever felt sad, lonely, bored, frustrated, or anxious and found yourself eating a candy bar, a bag of chips, fries, or a dish of ice cream to lift your spirits? A variety of foods can provide solace or comfort, and the choices depend on the individual. Many comfort foods are associated with a dish that a parent or caregiver prepared for you during early childhood. Maybe the comfort food is cookies with milk, bread pudding, macaroni and cheese, mashed potatoes, or some other simple dish.

Whatever the food, it may in some way brighten your mood. Thus eating becomes a quick antidote or a way to deal with negative emotions. Problems arise when comfort foods are high in calories and low in nutritional value. A person may be at risk for weight gain and unhealthy eating patterns, especially if eating becomes a habitual way of dealing with emotions.

Emotional eating is also prompted when people want to reward themselves for a job well done, a goal reached, or just because they think they deserve a treat. Maybe you want to celebrate an accomplishment, so you buy food and call your friends to "gather 'round the good stuff," which was once a slogan for a Pizza Hut commercial. Consuming food may also be a way to calm excitement or intense joy.

Health experts and dietitians recommend that people learn what emotions or circumstances trigger eating. Then instead of going for food immediately, a person should choose an alternative—go for a walk, listen to music, call a friend, or take part in an activity that has nothing to do with food.

Routine Eating

While our social networks and environment may contribute to unhealthy eating, personal habits also play a role and sometimes are entwined with environmental factors. Suppose someone always has a sweet snack after school or in the evening before bedtime. That could mean she or he has established an eating habit that might not be healthy. The same could be true if someone always has a high-calorie portion of popcorn when at the movies or watching TV at home.

Unhealthy eating may also be part of a person's daily lifestyle. A teenager on *Youth Radio Atlanta* put it this way:

> *I tell myself every day that I am going to eat healthy. But just the other morning, I ate a bag of potato chips for breakfast. That was a bad decision. There were many other healthier foods in my house but the chips were the easiest to eat and I was being lazy.*
>
> *I'm a little frightened about the effects of my diet later in life. The more garbage I eat, the more unhealthy my body becomes. And as I get older, I remind myself to eat salads, fresh fruits, and vegetables.*
>
> *Kids of my generation are eating so much junk food, it's going to be hard to convince everyone to change. I saw my friend pile on the pounds from eating lots of fast food and now I'm worried about her.*
>
> *I don't want to be one of those people who becomes heavy and then stays that way for the rest of their lives.*[5]

Another eating habit that can be a health risk is always having a breakfast, such as a cold cereal, that is primarily sugar. Some cereals contain more grams of sugar per serving than a chocolate bar. One more unhealthy habit is to sprinkle lots of sugar on unsweetened cereal. Eating breakfast tarts each morning is another example. The

Do You Know What to Eat?

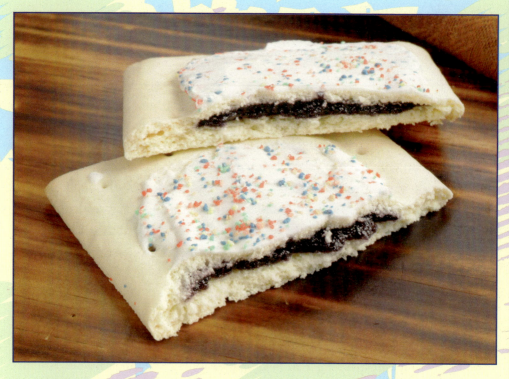

Sweet breakfasts may taste delicious, but their high sugar content is extremely unhealthy. In addition, they can make you want to eat larger portions because they don't contain fiber to make you feel full.

label on a box of raspberry Pop-Tarts shows that they contain several forms of sugar, such as dextrose and high fructose corn syrup, in the raspberry filling, as well as in the pastry itself. Donuts, sweet breads, pancakes and syrup, and white bread toast with jam or jelly are other examples of sugary breakfast items.

Breakfast with high sugar and low fiber content might cause people to overeat. After eating, blood sugar levels go up and then drop quickly so that a person craves more food later on. Ultimately this leads to weight gain.

The customary breakfast for Brittany, a young Utah teenager on the verge of being obese, was a Toaster Strudel with squeezable icing and Lucky Charms, a brand of cold cereal consisting of frosted oats

Our Eating Practices

and colored marshmallows. But in seventh grade she became aware that her breakfast was making her feel ill. "It happened after first period," Brittany told a reporter. "First, I couldn't see right, and then I'd get a huge migraine headache and throw up at school." As a result of feeling sick, Brittany would go home, miss classes, and have to make up the work. Her other eating habits were just as destructive. "I used to eat whatever I wanted," she said. "I would stuff myself until I was about to blow up."[6] She has changed to a healthy eating lifestyle by choosing salads, chicken, and fruit at the school cafeteria, eating small portions, and getting more exercise. And she is losing weight.

Skipping breakfast is another unhealthy habit, as numerous studies have shown, although some health experts contend that eating breakfast is not as crucial to health as once believed. Some people appear to benefit by having a daily breakfast; others do not. For example, many people omit breakfast as a means of losing weight, but that tactic does not necessarily work. Those who do not eat breakfast tend to get overly hungry later in the day and start consuming snacks or overeat at lunch or dinner. Avoiding breakfast also makes it difficult to get the vitamins and other nutrients the body needs daily.

Researchers at the Harvard School of Public Health conducted a study to determine whether skipping breakfast was a health risk. The results were published July 22, 2013 in the American Heart Association journal _Circulation_ and confirmed what has often been stated: breakfast is an important meal. "Skipping breakfast may lead to one or more risk factors, including obesity, high blood pressure, high cholesterol, and diabetes, which may in turn lead to a heart attack over time," the researchers concluded. [7]

Impacts on Eating Habits

Biology and family history can contribute to poor eating habits. Some studies have shown that even before a child is born, she or he may be programmed to prefer the taste of junk food if that is the mother's typical diet. Young people who grow up in a family whose

Do You Know What to Eat?

diet consists primarily of starches and few fruits and vegetables are likely to follow the same pattern.

Poverty may also play a major role, although low income does not necessarily indicate that members of a family will have unhealthy diets or tend to be overweight. In recent years, some studies have shown a link between poverty and obesity while others have shown that poverty has little or no impact on obesity. If low-income family members are obese, one of the reasons could be that the foods the family can afford are usually those that are filling but high in calories.

To help with food costs, the US Department of Agriculture maintains a Supplemental Nutrition Assistance Program (SNAP). Depending on monthly income, SNAP provides an allotment or payment in the form of an electronic debit card for households ranging in size from one to eight or more. For example, from September 2014 to October 2015, the allotment for a household of four was $649 per month; a household of eight received $1,169. [8]

But as the cost of food has been rising, it has become increasingly difficult to stretch food dollars to buy nutritious, low-calorie foods, such as fresh fruits and vegetables, fish, and lean meat. In addition, poor families may have limited access to nutritious foods, especially in inner-city neighborhoods where there are few if any supermarkets or fresh food stands.

Low-income urban families may also have to use public transportation to get to a major grocery store, and returning on a bus or subway with bags of groceries can be difficult. The alternative may be to shop at a neighborhood store that sells lots of junk foods or to eat at a fast food restaurant that offers large portions for a low price.

Yet healthy eating is possible even on an extremely limited budget. Advice on a healthy diet is available from numerous sources. But people may not take advantage of such resources if they do not understand how their eating habits may damage their health. Becoming aware of the effects of unhealthy eating is a first step toward changing to a nutritious dietary plan.

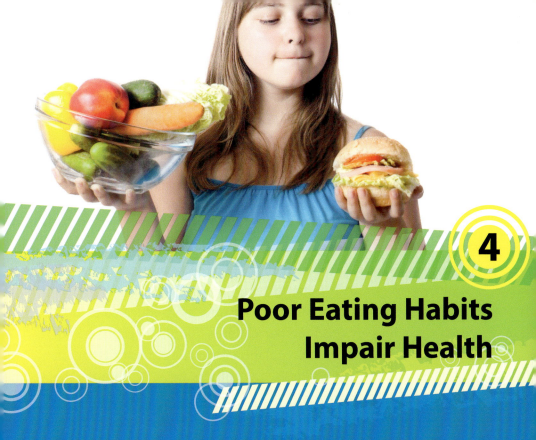

Poor Eating Habits Impair Health

Most of us eat without thinking a lot about whether our food will impair our health. After all, we need food to survive. But unhealthy eating can have harmful effects, which are publicized widely in the media, at schools, on Web sites, and elsewhere. So why do people eat foods that hurt them?

TV advertising and other promotions for junk food and food lacking in needed nutrients have helped encourage unhealthy eating habits among American young people, medical experts say. Junk foods and products with high sugar content appear in movies and video games, on clothing, toys, other merchandise, and almost any place where a logo or product image can be shown.

"On television alone the average US child sees approximately 13 food commercials every day, or 4,700 a year; and teens see more than 16 per day, or 5,900 in a year," according to a 2013 report from the Rudd Center for Food Policy and Obesity. "The food products advertised most extensively include high-sugar breakfast cereals, fast food and other restaurants, candy, and sugary drinks. In comparison, children see about one ad per week for healthy foods such as fruits and vegetables and bottled water." [1]

Because of the public concern about unhealthy eating patterns that can lead to being overweight and obesity among young people, some companies are taking part in the Children's Food and Beverage Advertising Initiative. Companies such as Campbell Soup, Coca-Cola, General Mills, Hershey, Kellogg, Kraft Foods, Mars, McDonald's, and PepsiCo have agreed to promote healthier products. In a 2012 issue of the journal *Childhood Obesity*, researchers advise communities to "become more educated on how food companies are reaching our children and the negative health consequences. Industry self-regulation has made modest changes in the foods marketed to children," the authors write. "Currently, the most promising strategy is to enact policies at the state and local level." These policies include prohibiting product labels on school property, as well as food advertising on school buses, and requiring "restaurants and stores to place only healthy items at kids' eye level; keeping unhealthy products like candy behind the counter." [2]

Obesity Rates and Effects

According to the US Centers for Disease Control and Prevention (CDC), "In 2012, more than one third of children and adolescents were overweight or obese. The percentage of children aged 6–11 years in the United States who were obese increased from 7% in 1980 to nearly 18% in 2012. Similarly, the percentage of adolescents aged 12–19 years who were obese increased from 5% to nearly 21% over the same period."

Obesity has both immediate and long-term effects on the health and well-being of young people, the CDC reports. Obese youth "are more likely to have risk factors for cardiovascular disease, such as high cholesterol or high blood pressure." They "are more likely to have prediabetes, a condition in which blood glucose levels indicate

Poor Eating Habits Impair Health

A Weighty Question

Besides the health problems linked to obesity, several early studies that were widely publicized suggested that overweight children are at greater risk of school absenteeism than their healthy-weight peers. In 2011, researchers analyzed records of students in grades one through twelve in Philadelphia, Pennsylvania, and concluded that "Obesity was weakly associated with increased school absences. . . . Overweight and obesity do not seem strongly associated with school absence, except among extremely obese children. Race and poverty appear to affect absences to a greater extent than overweight and obesity."[3]

Another study published in a 2012 issue of the *International Journal of Obesity* looked at absenteeism rates among 1,387 children aged six to eleven and 2,185 teens aged twelve to eighteen. The conclusion: "Increased body weight is independently associated with severe school absenteeism in children but not adolescents. Future research is needed to determine the nature and academic and social significance of this association."[4]

a high risk for development of diabetes" and "are at greater risk for bone and joint problems, sleep apnea, and social and psychological problems such as stigmatization and poor self-esteem." In the long term:

> Children and adolescents who are obese are likely to be obese as adults and are therefore more at risk for adult health problems such as heart disease, Type 2 diabetes, stroke, several types of cancer, and osteoarthritis. . . . Overweight and obesity are associated with increased risk for many types of cancer, including cancer of the breast, colon, endometrium, esophagus, kidney, pancreas, gall bladder, thyroid, ovary, cervix, and prostate, as well as multiple myeloma and Hodgkin's lymphoma.[5]

Do You Know What to Eat?

Diabetes—What It Is, Who Has It

Diabetes is a disease in which the body does not produce or properly use insulin, a hormone that converts glucose (sugar) and starch (such as potatoes) into energy the body cells need to function. There are two types of diabetes: Type 1 and Type 2. Type 1, once known as juvenile diabetes, is diagnosed in young people whose bodies do not produce insulin; they may need several insulin injections per day or an insulin pump to survive. Type 2 diabetes is the more common form. It develops gradually as a person's body fails to produce enough insulin or to use insulin efficiently. Type 2 diabetes used to be primarily an adult disease, but it has been rising steadily over the past decade in all children, especially African American, Hispanic, American Indian, and some Asian young people. Symptoms of diabetes include frequent urination, excessive thirst, extreme hunger, unusual weight loss, increased fatigue, irritability, and blurry vision.

While being overweight contributes to diabetes, other factors play a role, as well. Some people may be at risk for diabetes because the disease runs in their families. Although diabetes is not inherited, some people may be born with genes that make them prone to becoming diabetic. Studies are currently under way to determine whether or how genes may cause diabetes.

The American Diabetes Association (ADA) published "Data from the National Diabetes Statistics Report, 2014," which says that 29.1 million Americans, or 9.3 percent of the US population, had diabetes in 2012. That was an increase over 2010 when 25.8 million, or 8.3 percent, were diagnosed with diabetes. In 2012, 86 million Americans age twenty and older had prediabetes, up from 79 million in 2010. "About 208,000 Americans under age of twenty are estimated to have diagnosed diabetes," according to the report. The report lists percentages of people by racial and ethnic backgrounds who have diabetes. These are:

- 7.6% of non-Hispanic whites
- 9.0% of Asian Americans

Poor Eating Habits Impair Health

- 12.8% of Hispanics
- 13.2% of non-Hispanic blacks
- 15.9% of American Indians/Alaskan Natives [6]

Diabetes Facts and Fiction

Many people believe that diabetes is caused by eating too many sweets. Consuming sugary foods and beverages can lead to weight gain and can be a risk factor in developing diabetes. However, when eaten as part of a healthy meal plan or combined with exercise, sweets and desserts can be eaten in limited amounts by people with diabetes. The ADA has debunked other myths about diabetes. For example, some people believe diabetes is contagious. Diabetes is not an infection that you can catch like the flu.

The notion that people with diabetes should eat special diabetic foods is a myth. According to the ADA: "A healthy meal plan for people with diabetes is the same as that for everyone—low in fat (especially saturated and trans fat), moderate in salt and sugar, with meals based on whole grain foods, vegetables, and fruit. Diabetic and dietetic versions of sugar-containing foods offer no special benefit. They still raise blood glucose levels, are usually more expensive, and can also have a laxative effect if they contain sugar alcohols." [7]

There is a general belief that starchy foods, such as potatoes and pasta, are not good for diabetics. Yet as the ADA puts it, "Starchy foods can be part of a healthy meal plan, but portion size is key. Whole grain breads, cereals, pasta, rice, and starchy vegetables like potatoes, yams, peas and corn can be included in [diabetic] meals and snacks. In addition to these starchy foods, fruits, beans, milk, yogurt, and sweets are also sources of carbohydrates that you need to count in [a diabetic] meal plan." [8]

Other Problems Linked to Unhealthy Eating

Just as unhealthy eating can lead to obesity, it can also lead to heart disease and breathing problems. Heart disease includes heart attacks, high blood pressure, strokes, and atherosclerosis, or hardening of the

39

arteries. Atherosclerosis restricts the ability of blood vessels to carry oxygen and nutrients from a person's heart to the rest of her or his body. One risk factor for atherosclerosis is eating lots of saturated fat. Lack of exercise, smoking, and being overweight are other risk factors for developing atherosclerosis and other heart diseases.

Unhealthy eating also can lead to breathing problems, especially if a person is extremely overweight. The website livestrong.com puts it this way:

> Your weight can make a tremendous difference in how your respiratory system responds to environmental pollutants, as well as bacterial and viral assaults. When you are overweight, more of your body's energy is used to move, breathe, and complete daily tasks. This extra energy should be used in building and maintaining a healthy immune system. . . .
>
> By eating a balanced diet of carbohydrates, fats, and proteins, the body is better able to utilize what it needs through digestion and metabolism. When you eat too much of a single nutrient, the body utilizes more energy trying to regain that balance. According to the American Lung Association, carbohydrates produce more carbon dioxide than protein or fat. Therefore, a diet high in carbohydrates puts more stress on the respiratory system by requiring the lungs to release an abundance of carbon dioxide. [9]

Save Your Teeth!

As almost anyone who has been to a dentist knows, tooth decay occurs when plaque, a film of bacteria, stays on the teeth. The bacteria are fed by foods and beverages that contain sugar and starch, and they produce acids that can harm tooth enamel. When the harmful acids remain on the teeth, decay may result. Many people attempt to prevent this problem by brushing their teeth as frequently as possible.

Some eating habits can also have a detrimental effect on one's teeth. People who nibble on sugary snacks and sip soft drinks throughout the day may increase their risk of dental decay. Some

Poor Eating Habits Impair Health

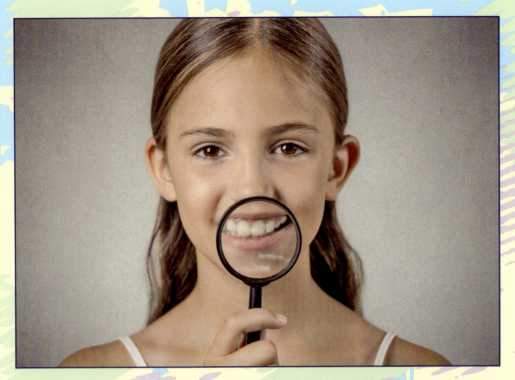

It is important to your overall health to take care of your teeth. Frequent brushing and daily flossing are essential for fighting decay, as are avoiding sugary drinks and snacks.

starchy foods, such as sweet breads and muffins, may also contain sugars, honey, molasses, or syrups that react with bacteria to produce acids. Even fresh or dried fruit with high sugar content (raisins, sweet cherries, berries, and oranges, for example) has the potential to cause cavities. Fruits that are firm and crunchy, such as apples and pears, are better choices for snacking because they are not as likely to cling to the surface of the teeth. Cough drops and mints can be culprits, too. They should be used sparingly because the sugar in them coats the teeth and acts just like candy to promote decay.

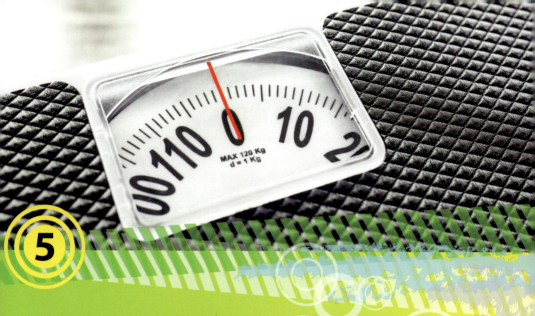

5

Dangerous Eating Behaviors

Many of the risks of unhealthy eating have already been described. But there are truly dangerous behaviors associated with eating. They are called eating disorders.

An eating disorder (ED) is a psychological condition that includes a distorted view of self and extreme disturbances in eating behavior. One ED is anorexia nervosa, usually known simply as anorexia; another is bulimia nervosa, or bulimia. Two other disorders are compulsive eating and binge eating.

The Eating Disorder Foundation describes these behaviors on its Web site:

> Anorexia nervosa is self-imposed starvation . . . a serious, life-threatening disorder, which usually stems from underlying emotional causes. Although people with anorexia nervosa are obsessed with food, they continually deny their hunger. People with anorexia nervosa often also limit or restrict other parts of

their lives besides food, including relationships, social activities, or pleasure. . . .

Bulimia nervosa . . . can be fatal if left untreated. People who have bulimia nervosa routinely "binge," consuming large amounts of food in a very short period of time, and immediately "purge," ridding their bodies of the just-eaten food by self-inducing vomiting, taking enemas, or abusing laxatives or other medications. . . .

People with compulsive overeating disorder suffer from episodes of uncontrolled eating or bingeing followed by periods of guilt and depression. Compulsive overeating is marked by the consumption of large amounts of food, sometimes accompanied by a pressured, "frenzied" feeling. Compulsive overeating disorder may cause a person to continue to eat even after they become uncomfortably full.

The essential features of binge-eating disorder are recurrent, out-of-control episodes of consuming abnormally large amounts of food. . . . Binge-eaters are usually extremely distressed by their eating behavior and experience feelings of disgust and guilt both during and after bingeing. [1]

Ron Saxen, a recovered binge eater, tells what it was like to gorge on food in his book *The Good Eater: The True Story of One Man's Struggle with Binge Eating Disorder*. Before overcoming his disorder, it was not unusual for him to consume "three Big Macs, a large order of fries, and a chocolate shake followed by four Hostess fruit pies, and a half gallon of Haagen-Dazs ice cream slathered with a pound of M&M's and a pint of hot fudge sauce."[2]

Usually, overeating creates guilt and even more stress and anxiety, so binge eaters repeat the practice, which creates a cycle of overeating. Binge eaters are likely to be overweight or obese.

Who Has Disturbed Eating Behaviors?

Studies conducted by government agencies, ED prevention organizations, and educational foundations measure the prevalence of eating disorders in the United States in different ways. Some

Do You Know What to Eat?

assess ED prevalence only among females, while others collect data on both females and males in all segments of society.

The University of Maryland Medical Center reported in 2013 that "about 7 million females and 1 million males suffer from eating disorders." These dangerous behaviors occur "most often in adolescents and young adults. They are also becoming increasingly prevalent among young children." The Center states "about 90-95% of patients with anorexia nervosa, and about 80% of patients with bulimia nervosa, are female. Most studies of individuals with eating disorders have focused on Caucasian middle-class females. However, eating disorders can affect people of all races and socioeconomic levels." [3]

What Can Cause an Eating Disorder

No one knows the exact causes of anorexia or bulimia, but one underlying factor is dissatisfaction with one's body. Females generally want to be thinner and males want to be more muscular than they actually are. Both genders are influenced by society's and the media's portrayals of what is supposed to be an ideal body.

Law Helps People with Eating Disorders

People with eating disorders often have mental health issues that require psychiatric counseling. But insurance plans may not cover psychiatric treatment for eating disorders. The Mental Health Parity and Addiction Equity Act of 2008 became effective in October 2010, and final rules were issued in November 2013. Basically, the rules say "patients with mental health and substance use disorders must be treated equally with medical/surgical benefits." That is, the rules require "equity with respect to financial requirements and treatment limitations under group health plans and group and individual health insurance coverage," according to the National Conference of State Legislatures. That means those who suffer EDs can be covered by health insurance. [4]

Dangerous Eating Behaviors

Girls and women are frequently obsessed with losing weight and want to look like fashion models or female celebrities with extremely thin figures. Advertising for clothes, cosmetics, and other beauty products feature images of picture-perfect models that girls and young women admire. They also want to be attractive to boys and men, who often believe that the ideal female body is like those portrayed in fashion advertisements. Females with EDs hope to achieve a skinny version of beauty even if it means being anorexic or bulimic.

Boys and men are also influenced by media images. They may resort to disordered eating to obtain the so-called ideal body type shown in advertisements for male cosmetics, hair and skin care, clothing, and other products. Males who are runners, dancers, jockeys, models, actors, entertainers, or in other professions requiring thinness frequently are particularly at risk for EDs.

A need to be in control is another major characteristic of people with disordered eating behavior. In order to feel in charge, they refuse to eat, or they purge themselves of food. They may express pride in having the willpower to resist food, and if they are tempted to eat something they like, they feel guilty. In some cases, a person with an ED may taste or chew food but spit it out before swallowing it.

EDs are coping skills, some experts say. Some people with eating disorders have been physically or sexually abused in their lives. They starve themselves into numbness so they will not have to feel the effects of disappointing and damaging relationships.

Another aspect of eating disorders is perfectionism. People with EDs may try to achieve nearly impossible goals. In school they try to get perfect grades, seek perfect relationships, and attempt to develop perfect bodies. Thus, in their view, they gain a sense of power. However, the feeling of power is an illusion. "Inside they feel weak, powerless, victimized, defeated, and resentful," according to the organization Anorexia Nervosa and Related Eating Disorders, Inc. (ANRED). On its Web site, ANRED points out:

Do You Know What to Eat?

> *People with eating disorders often lack a sense of identity. They try to define themselves by manufacturing a socially approved and admired exterior . . . by symbolically saying "I am, or I am trying to be, thin. Therefore, I matter."*
>
> *People with eating disorders often are legitimately angry, but because they seek approval and fear criticism, they do not dare express that anger directly. They do not know how to express it in healthy ways. They turn it against themselves by starving or stuffing.[5]*

Some of the theories that have been proposed regarding the causes of eating disorders include genetic factors. For some people, heredity plays a role in binge eating and the development of obesity. Brain chemistry may also be a factor. Imbalances in neurotransmitters, or nerve cells that send messages from one cell to another, may be responsible for anorexic behavior in some people.

How to Detect an Eating Disorder

While symptoms vary with individuals, people who have anorexia may diet, fast, or exercise excessively to lose pounds in spite of the

"Diabulimia"—It's Dangerous!

Another form of purging that is extremely dangerous is "diabulimia." The term comes from Type 1 diabetics, primarily teenage girls, who try to lose weight by not taking their needed insulin. Some diabetics with this disorder reason that insulin causes weight gain, so they can stay thin with smaller doses. Less insulin causes blood sugar to rise, and then a diabetic becomes very thirsty and drinks lots of water, urinating frequently. This gets rid of sugar and extra weight in the urine.

If blood sugar is not maintained in a healthy manner, a diabetic is at great risk for damage to the eyes, nerves, and kidneys. Blindness and heart failure can result. An immediate danger is a diabetic coma, which requires an emergency visit to the hospital.

Dangerous Eating Behaviors

fact that they already are at an abnormally low weight. If they do eat, they are likely to consume only a few foods in small amounts. They may weigh their food and count calories.

For newsplex.com, two teenagers, Victoria Lilly and Caroline Hazlett, described some of their anorexic symptoms and how they survived their eating disorder. "I never really had anything to talk about with any of my friends or anything because I was always preoccupied with food thoughts," Hazlett told reporter Loren Thomas. "People were always pushing like, 'You should eat, you should eat,' so then I didn't want to be with anyone," Lilly explained. She kept trying to lose weight and would "get to 115 pounds and be ok, then I wasn't. Then I was like, I'll get to 105 pounds and be okay, and then I was like no I need to lose more. . . . I just kept going and going."

"At her lowest weight, Victoria Lilly weighed only 80 pounds. Caroline Hazlett got down to an unhealthy weight as well. . . . Thanks to treatment and sessions with a nutritionist, both Caroline and Victoria are living healthy lives and have left their eating disorder in the past," Thomas reported.[6]

Like people with anorexia, those who have bulimia are obsessed with their weight. They may eat a large amount of food for a single meal and then immediately force themselves to vomit or use laxatives to get rid of what they consumed. This binge-purge cycle takes place on average fourteen times each week, experts say.

Warning signs that someone may have anorexia include dramatic weight loss over a short period of time, low body temperature (feeling cold much of the time), dry hair or skin, growth of baby-fine hair called lanugo on the body, swollen ankles and feet, fatigue, and in girls and women, cessation of menstrual periods. Signs of bulimia include erosion of tooth enamel from frequent vomiting, frequent trips to the bathroom, and use of laxatives or syrup of ipecac, which causes vomiting. People with eating disorders tend to exhibit some antisocial behaviors, such as avoiding events where food is served,

Do You Know What to Eat?

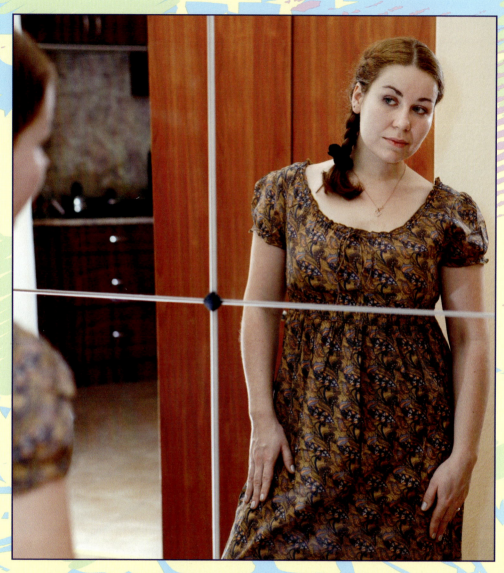

A person with an eating disorder may see something very different from her actual body when she looks in the mirror. She may stop eating because she believes her body image is too big.

refusing to eat with others, pretending to eat and throwing food away, and wearing oversized clothes to hide a thin body.

The binge-eating disorder is unlike bulimia in that people do not purge the food they eat. Symptoms may not be noticeable, except for weight gain, because binge eaters usually eat alone and may consume large amounts of food even though they do not feel hungry. Binge eating episodes are likely to occur several times per week.

Dangers to Health

There is no question that EDs can cause serious damage to a person's health and may be life threatening. One complication of anorexia is electrolyte imbalance. Electrolytes are essential for many bodily functions. They exist in the blood and include salts and minerals, such as sodium, calcium, potassium, chlorine, magnesium, and bicarbonate. Low levels of electrolytes can affect the body in many ways. Calcium deficiency, for example, can lead to low bone mass density. This can lead osteoporosis, a condition in which the bones become porous, which often results in bone fractures. Lack of potassium may result in muscle weakness, irritability, drowsiness, mental confusion, and irregular heartbeat.

Anorexia can also damage the heart, liver, and kidneys. Starvation slows down body functions and causes low blood pressure, pulse, and breathing rate. As a result, an anorexic person may be light-headed and unable to concentrate. Depression is also common among anorexics, which sometimes leads to suicide. The risk of heart problems is ever present, which can be life threatening. In short, anorexia can kill.

Some researchers say that between 5 and 20 percent of those with anorexia die from the disorder. As ANRED puts it: "Without treatment, up to twenty percent (20%) of people with serious eating disorders die. With treatment, that number falls to two to three percent (2–3%)."[7]

Do You Know What to Eat?

The damaging effects of bulimia include stomach pain and tooth decay from acids in the mouth due to vomiting. Because people with bulimia throw up frequently, their salivary glands may expand, which creates "chipmunk" cheeks. Purging through vomiting or laxative use can also cause potassium loss and dehydration.

People with EDs may resort to excessive exercise to lose weight. While exercise is important for good health, compulsive exercise could be a sign of an ED. Some may spend hours each day lifting weights, doing sit-ups, riding stationary bikes, and using treadmills and other exercise equipment. Or they may run miles every day and wear heavy sweats over plastic wraps to increase perspiration and lose water weight. Excessive exercise can cause bone fractures and muscle strains.

The consequences of binge eating can be just as serious than the effects of anorexia or bulimia. Binge eating can cause or be closely linked to obesity, diabetes, heart disease, high blood pressure, and stroke.

While health experts continue to warn about disordered eating, they also consistently urge people with EDs to find help. Numerous organizations are available for that purpose. ANRED is one; another is the National Association of Anorexia Nervosa and Associated Disorders (ANAD). Others include the National Eating Disorders Association, American Anorexia/Bulimia Association, Harvard Eating Disorders Center, and many local ED clinics, camps, and support groups. People who recover from disordered eating learn how to cope with their psychological condition and to eat in healthy ways.

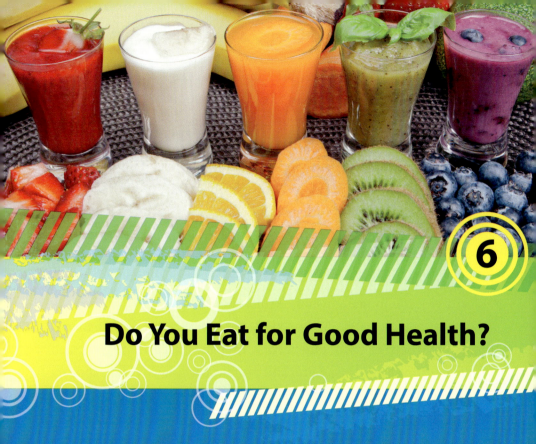

Do You Eat for Good Health?

No doubt you have read or heard about healthy eating. Messages about what you should eat for good health seem to come at you from many directions—at medical offices, school, or home, on TV and videos, in grocery stores, and even in comic books.

For years, food guides in the United States have been provided by government agencies to educate people about healthy food choices. Dietitians, nutritionists, and medical experts also offer advice on healthy eating. So does the media. In other words, there is an abundance of information, and most of it is based on the *Dietary Guidelines for Americans* produced by the US Department of Health and Human Services (DHHS) and the USDA. The guidelines are online and include a chapter on "Building Healthy Eating Patterns."[1] In addition, the USDA's MyPlate is frequently used as a basis for how to eat in a healthful manner.

Do You Know What to Eat?

The current version of the USDA MyPlate shows the recommended food groups and their proportional amounts. A poster titled "What's On Your Plate?" at www.choosemyplate.gov shows healthy choices. Half the plate should contain fruits and vegetables, shown in red and green respectively. The other half indicates grains in brown and protein in purple. On the side is a small blue plate representing dairy foods.

Below the graphic of the plate are suggestions for the various choices. For example, under vegetables instructions say, "Eat more red, orange, and dark green veggies like tomatoes, sweet potatoes, and broccoli in main dishes." Fruits should be chosen for, "snacks, salads, and desserts. At breakfast, top your cereal with bananas or strawberries; add blueberries to pancakes." There are also suggestions for grains, dairy, and protein choices. MyPlate appears on a Web site that also includes The SuperTracker, which can help you plan, analyze, and track your diet and physical activity.[2]

However, the Harvard School of Public Health takes issue with some of the USDA recommendations. In 2011, the School of Public Health and Harvard Health Publications released its guide for nutritious meals. Called Healthy Eating Plate, it has a graphic similar to MyPlate, and "specifies that consumers should stick to whole grains instead of refined grains, eat healthy proteins such as fish or poultry rather than red or processed meats, and distinguish between healthy vegetables and potatoes." The Harvard plan "also includes a glass of water and healthy oils in its ideal meal, advising consumers to avoid butter and trans fat." According to Professor Willett, a nutrition expert at Harvard, "The intent [with Healthy Eating Plate] is to make an eating guide based on the best available scientific evidence and to provide consumers with the information that they need to make choices that can profoundly affect their health and well-being."[3]

The Harvard School's website says the USDA's guidelines are:

Do You Eat for Good Health?

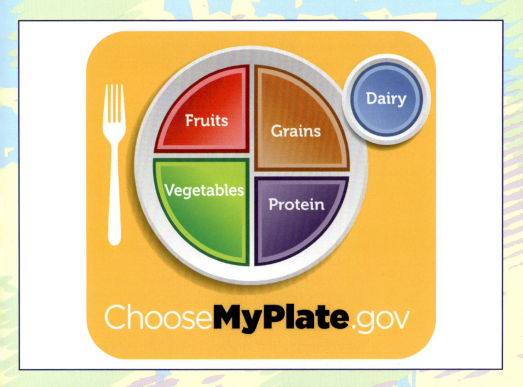

This handy graphic from the USDA illustrates how each meal should be broken down. Fruits and vegetables should share your plate equally with grains and protein. How does your plate compare?

Too lenient on red meat. The guidelines still continue to lump red meat together with fish, poultry, eggs, nuts, seeds, beans, and soy products in one food group, newly termed the 'protein foods' group. Though they highlight the benefits of replacing some meat or chicken with fish, they gloss over the substantial evidence that replacing red meat with poultry, beans, or nuts could help prevent heart disease and that lowering red meat can lower the risk of diabetes.

Another criticism is the recommendation to increase:

the intake of low-fat milk and dairy products.... There is little, if any, evidence that eating dairy prevents osteoporosis or fractures, and there is considerable evidence that high dairy product

Do You Know What to Eat?

> consumption is associated with increased risk of fatal prostate and ovarian cancers. To be sure, calcium is an important nutrient, but we don't need as much calcium as these guidelines recommend— and milk and dairy are not the only, or best, sources of calcium.[4]

Healthier School Foods

Because of concerns about the harmful health effects of junk food, schools across the United States have been replacing candy, chips, and sugary soft drinks with nutritious food and beverage items in vending machines. Similar changes have been taking place in school cafeterias.

To decrease overall consumption of junk foods among students, a USDA policy called Smart Snacks in School was prompted by the Healthy, Hunger-Free Kids Act of 2010. That act requires the USDA to establish nutrition standards for all foods sold in schools. "The Smart Snacks in School regulation applies to foods sold a la carte, in the school store, and vending machines. Prior to the publishing of the Smart Snacks rule, 39 states already had nutrition standards in place," the USDA said.[5]

Most states now mandate that their school vending machines offer healthy alternatives to such snacks as candy bars, sugary sodas, and fried chips. Water, sports drinks, juice, granola bars, and baked chips are some items offered instead. School cafeterias also help students make healthful food choices. As part of the Healthy, Hunger-Free Kids Act, the USDA attempted to limit the amount of french fries to no more than two servings a week in school lunches. But Congress did not go along and said there should be no limits on any vegetables. Pizza was also kept on the school lunch menu because tomato sauce is considered a vegetable, although it cannot be the only one. A side of another vegetable has to be included, and the crust must be made with whole grains and low in sodium.

What about free school lunches operated by the National School Lunch Program? Schools that take part in the program receive cash subsidies for meals and USDA surplus foods. The program operates

Do You Eat for Good Health?

in one hundred thousand public schools, nonprofit private schools, and residential child care institutions, which serve "more than 31 million children each school day in 2012." Do all those meals contain healthy foods?

According to the program's fact sheet:

> School lunches must meet meal pattern and nutrition standards based on the latest Dietary Guidelines for Americans. The current meal pattern increases the availability of fruits, vegetables, and whole grains in the school menu. . . While school lunches must meet Federal meal requirements, decisions about what specific foods to serve and how they are prepared are made by local school food authorities.[6]

Some colleges report that over the past few years there has been an increase in the number of students requesting and buying healthy foods. Food service directors are adding low-calorie, low-fat, and low-carbohydrate items, as well as vegetarian options, for students. Food stations with salads and fruits are also available. At the University of California Irvine, a Healthy Heart station features a complete meal that is fewer than five hundred calories, contains no trans fat, is low in salt, low in cholesterol, and sugar free.

Along with serving healthy meals, some universities have promoted ways to help students incorporate green vegetables into their diets. Students, for example, may learn how to eat green foods, such as spinach omelets, at breakfast. A promotional effort at Johns Hopkins University in Maryland highlighted vegetarian cooking with a dining services chef demonstrating how to prepare a healthful vegetarian meal in a simple and efficient way.

Dining Services at the University of Connecticut supports and promotes a Local Routes program, the goal of which is to use local foods in its food service operations. A student-run EcoGarden near campus works with Local Routes to supply produce for the university's Whitney Dining Hall, where vegetarian and vegan meals are served. Local farms provide other foods, such as various cheeses

Do You Know What to Eat?

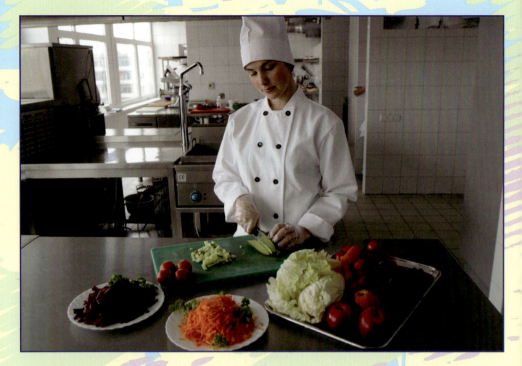

The government has pushed school cafeterias to offer healthier food options for students. Incorporating more vegetables into your favorite meals is an easy way to start.

from the Calabro Cheese Company in East Haven, Connecticut, and apples, pears, peaches, and apple cider from Buell's Orchard in Eastford, Connecticut. Maple syrup, beef hotdogs, and tofu are some other items from local sources.[7]

How to Shop for Healthy Food

Grocery stores are attempting to do their part to encourage healthy eating. Numerous stores provide information about the nutrient content of fresh vegetables and fruits either on charts or on produce shelves or bins. Fresh produce, whole grain breads, meats, seafood, and dairy products are on the perimeter of most large stores. So if a shopper wants to fill a cart with fresh food, the place to start is on the outer edges of the store.

Do You Eat for Good Health?

When shopping for canned, frozen, or other packaged foods, the source for nutrient content is the information panel called the nutrition facts label, which as described previously, shows the serving size and how many calories there are per serving. The label also indicates the total amount of fat with a breakdown of saturated, polyunsaturated, monounsaturated, and trans fat, cholesterol, certain vitamins and minerals by percentage of daily value (%DV)— the recommended daily allowance for a nutrient based on a 2,000 calorie diet—sodium (salt), protein, sugar, and fiber content.

Ingredients on the label are listed beginning with the greatest amount to the least. Consider sugar and other forms of sugar, which include dextrose, fructose, high fructose corn syrup, fruit juice concentrates, honey, and molasses. If these sweeteners are high on the list, as they often are on the labels for cold cereal, pastries, and other processed foods, you may want to find a less sugary product and one that may be lower in calories and higher in nutrients.

The packaging on some food items may declare that a product has 50 percent less fat or half the salt. These can be meaningless terms unless a person knows what the product is being compared with—is it 50 percent of the same type and quantity of product? For example, a package of turkey bacon says that it has 65 percent less fat than pork bacon, so to truly compare, a person would have to know the amount of fat in both kinds of bacon. A label on a store brand of canned corn says 50 percent less salt, but it does not make a comparison with anything. However, the label likely means that can of corn has half the salt of the store's regular brand of canned corn. A quick check of the nutrition facts on both the regular and low-salt store brand of canned corn shows the regular canned corn contains 310 milligrams of sodium and the other contains 150 milligrams of sodium—50 percent less salt than the regular canned corn.

Health and nutrition assertions are a different story. The federal Nutrition Labeling and Education Act requires that certain food claims abide by explicit rules. If the term free is used, the product must contain no amount or only trivial amounts of a specific

Do You Know What to Eat?

ingredient. The terms sugar free and fat free, for example, mean less than 0.5 grams of sugar or fat per serving. If a low fat claim is made, the product must have no more than 3 grams of fat per serving. Low sodium means fewer than 140 milligrams of salt per serving, very low sodium is 35 milligrams or less per serving, and sodium free means less than 0.5 milligrams of salt. One serving of a low calorie product must contain no more than 40 calories.

To help grocery shoppers choose healthy foods, the AHA created a heart-check symbol, which certifies that the product with the red heart and white check mark is low in saturated fat and cholesterol. However, the AHA cautions that its certification program is designed for healthy people and anyone with a medical condition should see a physician or dietitian before making changes to her or his diet.

Anyone with access to the Internet can create a personalized heart-healthy grocery list online from more than eight hundred foods listed as low in saturated fat and cholesterol on the AHA Web site. Choices can be made by food type or manufacturer. Once products are selected, a list can be printed to take along to the store.

Shopping Challenges

For families with a limited income, it is not easy to buy healthy food. Millions of low-income families get help with the SNAP program funded by the federal government. Depending on a family's monthly benefit, an individual has about $4.40 per day for meals. In 2013, twenty-six members of Congress participated in the SNAP Challenge, a program first called the Food Stamp Challenge that began nationally in 2007 to illustrate the difficulties of trying to buy nutritious food and drinks for a few dollars per day.

US Representative Barbara Lee (D-CA) took part in the first challenge and has been promoting it ever since. In 2007, she had about $3.00 per day for food. She reported that one day she "had grits and toast for breakfast, crackers and a banana for lunch, and two hamburgers from White Castle ($.51 apiece) for dinner." Another day, she found a discount grocery store to buy "a small container of

Do You Eat for Good Health?

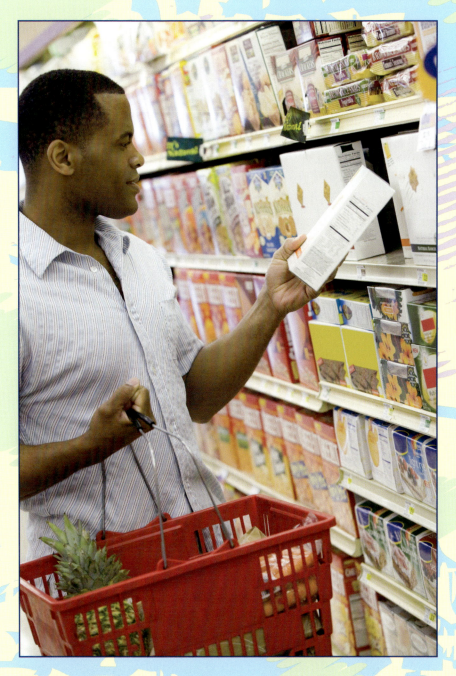

Grocery stores offer an abundance of products promising health benefits. Learn to ignore the claims on the box and make your own decisions based on nutrition labels.

Do You Know What to Eat?

chicken and dumplings, an apple, a can of tuna, a box of macaroni and cheese, and a can of turnip greens (total $2.25)." By the middle of the week, she reported: "It's hard to concentrate for any length of time on anything except food. I don't know how people with no money for decent meals do anything—study, work, exercise, read, have fun, etc. It's all about just making it through the day."[8]

Six years later Lee was one of the participating members who tried to buy a week's groceries for about $30.00, or a daily stipend of a little more than $4.00 for food and beverages. She could not buy butter and milk—they were too expensive. In a blog post, she wrote:

> First, I went straight for the crackers. They're cheap, they last a long time, and they're portable. . . . Next, I find canned tuna, canned peas, and a box to make tuna noodle casserole. . .that will last several days and is fairly balanced. Beyond that, I find eggs with six to a carton, not 12, which is helpful, as well as a sale on yams, and get one for $.49/lb. . . . I made sure to add an apple (the smallest one in the bunch, they're calculated by the pound), a small onion, and a can of lima beans. I try hard to get some more fresh fruit and vegetables, but they're out of my price range. Canned vegetables have too much sodium, but they're cheap. Canned fruits have too much sugar, but they're cheap. Shopping carts can be filled with good, nutritious food if you have the money for it. If not, you have a recipe for diabetes and hypertension on your hands. . . .
>
> What I'm thinking about most during this trip is that I'm shopping only for myself. When I was a young, single mother, I was on public assistance. It was a bridge over troubled water, and without it, I wouldn't be where I am today. I spent hours debating what to buy and what to skip, all the while keeping my sons in my mind. I could go without breakfast; my sons couldn't.[9]

In spite of the problems of eating healthfully on a tight budget, planning carefully is an important element, as Congresswoman Lee pointed out. Other money-saving suggestions include stocking up on staples, such as beans, brown rice, pasta, oatmeal, and barley,

Do You Eat for Good Health?

when available at a low price. These can stretch soups, stews, and casseroles and add fiber. Using store coupons saves on grocery bills, as does shopping for produce in season and for sale items in the canned and frozen-food sections.

Ads Determine Food and Beverage Choices

Whether or not cost is a factor in grocery shopping, healthy eating means being aware of how advertising on television, YouTube, Facebook, Twitter, MySpace, and other social media affects food choices. If young children go along to the grocery store, they frequently beg for products such as sugary cereals and high-calorie snacks endorsed by their favorite cartoon characters. Teenagers also are influenced to buy food and beverage products touted in the media.

Nevertheless, some changes have taken place. In June 2012, Disney became the first major media company to apply nutrition standards for ads placed on TV programs directed to children. Cartoon Network followed that example. The companies prohibit the use of their commercial characters to promote foods and beverages high in fat, calories, and sugar. Instead, advertised items must meet specific limits for these ingredients.

Food and beverage companies are also on board with changes in their advertising directed at children. Burger King, Campbell Soup, Coca-Cola, General Mills, Hershey, Kellogg, Kraft Foods, Mars, McDonald's, PepsiCo, and Unilever are taking part in the Children's Food and Beverage Advertising Initiative. These companies have agreed to promote healthier products. The Council of Better Business Bureaus monitors whether companies are complying with the initiative's guidelines.

Currently, it is debatable whether the marketing strategy to limit unhealthy food and beverage ads aimed at children and teens will be successful. The fact remains that hundreds of commercials for foods and beverages with little nutrient value are aired daily in the media and can influence viewers, no matter what their age group.

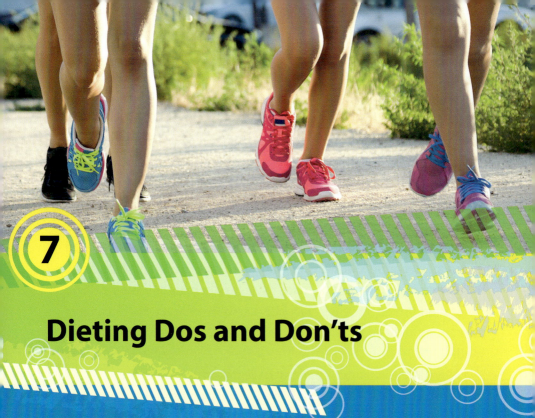

7

Dieting Dos and Don'ts

Americans are bombarded by claims that a particular diet will assure weight loss. Healthy eating involves a daily diet that provides adequate nutrients and helps a person maintain an appropriate weight. But many people who want to lose pounds turn to weight-loss diets and diet pills, which can be expensive, ineffective, and even dangerous. Teenagers are sometimes especially concerned about their body image and are likely to try the latest diet advertised. Their goal is to achieve the perfect weight, and they risk engaging in disordered eating behaviors.

According to one study of more than twenty-five hundred junior high and high school students, girls in middle school who read dieting articles were twice as likely to try to lose weight compared to girls who never read such articles. The researchers concluded:

Frequent reading of magazine articles about dieting and weight-loss strongly predicted unhealthy weight-control behaviors in adolescent girls, but not boys. . . . Findings from this study, in conjunction with findings from previous studies, suggest a need for interventions aimed at reducing exposure to, and the importance placed on, media messages regarding dieting and weight loss.[1]

Choosing a Weight-Loss Diet

Anyone who has ever done a search on the Internet to find information about weight-loss diets knows that thousands of hits appear. Millions of people look for a quick fix to their weight problems. The Paleo or Caveman diet is a popular choice. That diet recommends eating fresh lean meats and fish, fruits, vegetables, and healthy fats. Eggs, nuts, and seeds also are included. On that diet, people are advised to avoid dairy products, refined sugar, potatoes, salt, and refined vegetable oils, such as canola.

Some dieters choose all-liquid diet plans that focus on drinking protein drinks, tea, apple cider vinegar, or other liquids while eliminating other foods. Or they might try diets that call for eating primarily a single food, such as the Grapefruit Diet or the Cabbage Soup Diet. Grapefruit can help curb appetite before a meal or it can be a nutritious snack, but it has no special qualities to burn off fat. Cabbage soup can be a healthy meal, but eating it for most meals can cause bloating and gas. In short, neither all-liquid diets nor single-food diets are nutritionally sound.

Some weight-loss diets include low-carbohydrate (low-carb) and high-protein diets, such as the Atkins Diet, South Beach Diet, and the Zone Diet. The Atkins Diet is one of the most widely used low-carb diets. The diet severely limits high-carb foods, such as breads, pasta, fruits, sugar, and some vegetables. But the diet allows unlimited amounts of protein.

Ever since it was initiated in the 1970s, the Atkins Diet has been controversial. Some health experts consider the diet dangerous because it limits carbohydrates the body needs and allows protein foods that are high in saturated fats, which increases the risk of heart disease and obesity. People on the Atkins Diet may lose weight

Do You Know What to Eat?

quickly in the short term because they lose water at first, but over the long term, Atkins dieters lose no more weight than people on a low-fat, low-calorie diet, some researchers say.

Among the popular diets are detox diets that promise quick weight loss and disease prevention by supposedly cleansing the body of toxins or poisons. Hundreds of books and magazine articles tout these diet plans, which are based on the premise that we take in many toxic materials in foods and chemicals in our environment and that we need to remove these poisons from our bodies. Certain foods and liquids are supposed to detoxify and not only reduce pounds but also offer benefits ranging from increased energy to reversal of cancer.

Detox diets frequently begin with fasting for a few days and then extremely limit foods or require a liquid diet of various concoctions, such as one made of lemon juice, maple syrup, water, and cayenne pepper. Laxatives may also be part of the regimen, which can last from a week to ten days.

Health experts warn against such diets. The Mayo Clinic, for example, says: "there's little evidence that detox diets actually remove toxins from the body. Indeed, the kidneys and liver effectively filter and eliminate most ingested toxins. The benefits from a detox diet may actually come from avoiding highly processed foods that have solid fats and added sugar." [2]

Teenagers need to be especially cautious about detox plans or any severe food restrictions or long fasts. Detox diets lack the nutrients that teens require for their growth and development. Athletes and teens involved in daily physical activities require enough food for energy; fasting and detox diets do not provide the needed calories.

The American Heart Association puts it this way:

> *Quick weight-loss diets usually overemphasize one particular food or type of food. They violate the first principle of good nutrition: Eat a balanced diet that includes a variety of foods. If you are able to stay on a quick weight-loss diet for more than a few weeks, you may develop nutritional deficiencies, because no one type of food*

has all the nutrients you need for good health. . . . There are no "superfoods." That's why you should eat moderate amounts from all food groups, not large amounts of a few special foods. These diets also violate a second important principle of good nutrition: Eating should be enjoyable. These diets are so monotonous and boring that it's almost impossible to stay on them for long periods.[3]

Some diet programs do encourage a variety of healthy food choices. Two examples are Weight Watchers and the Jenny Craig Diet Program. There are few if any forbidden foods, but dieters are advised to limit calories. Both programs have support systems to help dieters establish and maintain a healthy eating pattern.

Whatever the weight-loss diets, they are usually widely advertised—on TV, the Internet, billboards, and in the print media. Their claims should be looked at critically. They may be suspect if they state that a dieter will lose more than one or two pounds per week, if they promise weight loss on a continual basis without exercising, if they limit food choices and do not offer a balanced diet that meets nutritional needs, if they say their product has been tested by a respected or leading medical center or university but provide no information on who, where, and how the study was conducted, or if they present testimonials from clients or experts who might be paid for their endorsements. To be safe, advice about a weight-loss diet should come from your family doctor, nurse, reputable nutritionist, dietitian, or health organization. In short, "the only sensible way to lose weight and maintain a healthy weight permanently is to eat less and balance your food intake with physical activity," as the AHA points out.[4]

Some Dangers of Diet Pills

Diet pills and herbal supplements may pose risks to people trying to lose weight. Among the risk takers are young teenagers. One study conducted over a five-year period found that 20 percent of the females surveyed had used diet pills by the age of twenty. "Diet pills are not safe for teen use. For one thing, diet pills may contain a variety

Do You Know What to Eat?

Facts About Losing Weight

Many nutritionists, government agencies, and health organizations have warned consumers about dieting myths by countering them with factual information. Some of these are below:

Myth: Quick weight-loss diets result in permanent weight loss.
Fact: It is possible to lose weight at first, but diets that limit food choices may result in lost nutrients the body needs.

Myth: High-protein/low-carbohydrate diets are a healthy way to lose weight.
Fact: The long-term health effects of such diets are unknown.

Myth: Starches are fattening and should be limited when trying to lose weight.
Fact: Many starchy foods are low in fat and calories and an important source of energy, but if eaten in large portions and with toppings like butter and cheese they can become high in fat and calories.

Myth: Certain foods can help burn fat and lose weight.
Fact: No foods can burn fat.

Myth: Natural or herbal weight-loss products are safe and effective.
Fact: Such products usually are not scientifically tested for safety or effectiveness.

Myth: People can lose weight by eating whatever they want.
Fact: To lose weight, a person should limit the calories and portions of the foods they eat.

Myth: People can lose weight by not eating.
Fact: Anyone who starves can lose pounds but will also lose nutrients and muscle mass; pounds will return when a person starts eating again.

Myth: Fast foods are always an unhealthy choice for dieters.
Fact: Fast foods can be part of a diet plan if a person carefully selects small portions of low-calorie items.

of harmful chemicals, such as ephedrine or phenylpropranolamine, which can have powerful stimulant effects on teens," writes Natalie Smith on livestrong.com. "Many diet pills are addictive and can lead to other serious consequences for health in the long term such as insomnia, high blood pressure, or even death if the teen uses the pills incorrectly or over a long period of time."[5]

According to the Mayo Clinic, most weight-loss pills are "probably ineffective" or there is "insufficient evidence to evaluate them." Many decrease appetite but have no proven ability to reduce a person's weight and may cause gastrointestinal or other problems.[6]

The FDA regulates dietary supplements under a different set of rules than those covering conventional foods and over the counter (OTC) drugs. "Although dietary supplement manufacturers must register their facilities with FDA, they are not required to get FDA approval before producing or selling dietary supplements. Manufacturers and distributors must make sure that all claims and information on the product label and in other labeling are truthful and not misleading." In addition, the FDA says "the manufacturer, packer, or distributor whose name appears on the label of a dietary supplement marketed in the United States is required to submit to [the] FDA all serious adverse event reports associated with use of the dietary supplement in the United States."[7] Weight-loss aids may be labeled as supplements so that manufacturers can make health claims about their products based on their own reviews and interpretations of studies without the authorization of the FDA.

Some products contain ephedra, also known as ma huang, a traditional Chinese medicine that acts like amphetamines, or uppers. In 2004, the FDA banned ephedra, but it is still available for sale on the Internet and in some stores. What the FDA actually banned was "alkaloids of ephedrine, found mainly in the stem of the ephedra. . . . It's the chemical presumably responsible for weight loss but also for boosting heart rate and blood pressure," according to *Consumer Reports* magazine. However, extracts "that contain little or no ephedrine" are legal and "aren't likely to pose dangers."[8]

Do You Know What to Eat?

Like advertising for weight-loss diets, claims about the effectiveness of diet pills and supplements can be misleading or fraudulent. Benjamin Plackett, a contributor to *Inside Science*, wrote in 2013, "Researchers at Dartmouth College, in N.H., and the University of Wisconsin-Madison decided to check up on what drug companies say in their US TV commercials. Their findings suggest a frequent disregard for the truth. Sixty percent of prescription drug ads and 80 percent of over the counter drug ads were found to be misleading or false." [9]

Calorie Content on Restaurant Menus

Although many fast food restaurants advertise or promote low-calorie items on their menus, that does not mean that a total meal will actually have low caloric content. Customers frequently forget the calories in side dishes or soft drinks that they order. In an exploratory study in 2013 to evaluate the effect of menu labeling on fast food menu offerings, CDC researchers found that, "Beginning with New York City in 2008, 18 states and localities have implemented regulations requiring chain restaurants to post calorie information on menus and menu boards. . . . Although it is too early to assess the full impact of menu labeling on consumer choice, research to date has shown mixed results." The researchers concluded that "menu labeling has thus far not affected the average nutritional content of fast food menu items, but it may motivate restaurants to increase the availability of healthier options." [10]

When New York City's calorie labeling regulation was being considered, the state's Restaurant Association challenged the ordinance by declaring it was too expensive to implement and would do little if anything to prevent people from eating foods high in calories. Other critics argued that it was not the responsibility of any government to see that people eat healthfully. In their view, that amounted to a nanny state—having someone constantly watching over the public and interfering with free choice.

Dieting Dos and Don'ts

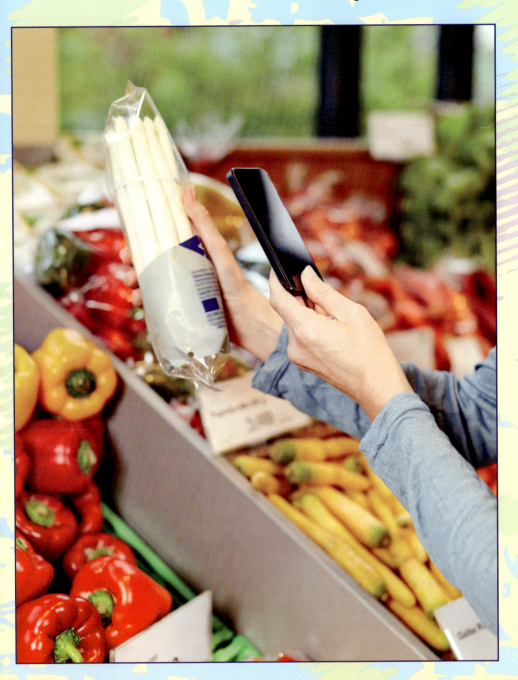

Spartphones are a helpful tool when trying to eat healthfully. There are plenty of apps available that can provide you with calorie counts, recipes, nutritional benefits, and other information.

Do You Know What to Eat?

Supporting the legislation were Public Citizen and the Center for Science in the Public Interest plus prominent health organizations, nutrition professors, and government officials. According to Public Citizen:

> *American adults and children consume about one third of their calories from restaurants and other food-service establishments, and studies link frequent eating out with obesity and higher caloric intakes. Without nutrition information, it is difficult for consumers to make informed choices. In requiring fast food restaurants to disclose calorie information on their menus, New York City has taken the lead in addressing one of the largest contributors to the nation's obesity epidemic.[11]*

Serving Size

Even if you are able to check out the calories and nutrients in restaurant food, the information may not help much if you do not control the portions you eat. Whether we eat out or at home, most of us misjudge the amount of food or beverage we consume, which can easily result in taking in more calories than expected.

Some restaurant menus and all packaged, canned, or bottled groceries show serving sizes, which vary depending on the item. But how do you determine a serving size? The Weight-control Information Network explains,

> *A serving size is the amount of food listed on a product's food label, and it varies from product to product. A portion is how much food you choose to eat at one time, whether in a restaurant, from a package, or at home. Sometimes the serving size and portion size match; sometimes they do not.*
>
> *For example, according to a food label, one cup of macaroni and cheese is one serving. But if you make yourself a large bowl of macaroni and cheese, that portion is much bigger than one serving. The same may be true if you pour yourself a large bowl of cereal for breakfast. You should be the judge of how the portion*

Dieting Dos and Don'ts

you choose to eat relates to the serving size noted on the food label.[12]

When you are away from home and do not have any kind of measurement tool, how do you determine portions? Sometimes it helps to compare the amount of food with everyday objects:

- 3 ounces (85 g) of meat or poultry = a deck of cards
- 1 cup or 8 fl oz (227 g) of cereal = a fist
- 1/2 cup or 4 oz (113 g) of cooked rice, pasta, or potato = 1/2 baseball
- 1 baked potato = a fist
- 1 medium fruit = a baseball
- 1/2 cup or 4 oz (113 g) of fresh fruit = 1/2 baseball
- 1 1/2 ounces (43 g) of low-fat or fat-free cheese = 4 stacked dice
- 1/2 cup or 4 fl oz (113 ml) of ice cream = 1/2 baseball
- 2 tablespoons (30 g) of peanut butter = a ping-pong ball

Another way to control portions when eating out is to order a small children's-size meal, or before you start eating, ask for a take-home box to save half your meal. Eating a salad before lunch or dinner can help curb appetite and the temptation to eat a large meal. One more tip is to stop eating when you begin to feel full. Finally, no fad diet or pill is a substitute for nutritious foods in sensible portions to reach and stay at a healthy weight.

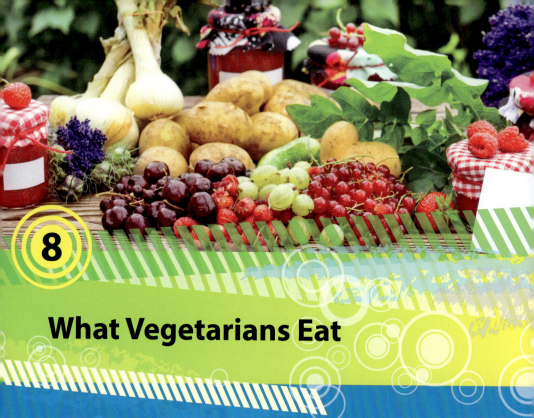

8

What Vegetarians Eat

Vegetarians do not eat meat, fish, or poultry, but along with plant foods, they eat eggs, milk, and dairy products, such as cheese and yogurt. Some people consider themselves semi-vegetarians—they do not eat red meat but include chicken and fish with plant foods, dairy products, and eggs.

Because a vegan diet does not include animal products, protein, vitamin B-12, vitamin D, iron, and calcium may be in short supply. But there are alternatives to animal products. Protein is found in soybeans, legumes, nuts, seeds, and whole grains. Enriched cereals and fortified soy contain B-12, which is needed by red blood cells. Iron is also an essential component of red blood cells and can be found in dark green vegetables (broccoli, romaine lettuce, and other leafy greens), dried beans and peas, lentils, and whole grain products.

What Vegetarians Eat

Lacto and lacto-ovo vegetarians obtain their protein and calcium from dairy products. Other major protein sources include beans, nuts, and soy products. For lacto-ovos, eggs are a protein source, as well.

Choosing a Vegetarian Diet

Going vegetarian is an option that an increasing number of teenagers and preteens are choosing. Although only a minority of teens make such a choice, parents, public health officials, school personnel, and others frequently ask if a vegetarian diet is healthy. Answers come from many quarters. As might be expected, vegetarian groups highly endorse such a diet. Some medical groups do also, but with cautionary notes. The American Heart Association, for example, says:

> *Many studies have shown that vegetarians seem to have a lower risk of obesity, coronary heart disease (which causes heart attack), high blood pressure, diabetes mellitus, and some forms of cancer. Vegetarian diets can be healthful and nutritionally sound if they're carefully planned to include essential nutrients. However, a vegetarian diet can be unhealthy if it contains too many calories and not enough important nutrients.[1]*

A research report in the *Journal of Pediatric Health Care* noted: "Many well-designed studies have concluded that children and adolescents who follow a properly designed vegetarian diet grow and develop normally." In addition, the report states:

> *Research has highlighted nutritional advantages to vegetarian diets and has indicated that this style of eating can lead to lifelong healthy eating habits when adopted at a young age. Studies show that children and adolescents who follow a vegetarian diet have a lower intake of cholesterol, saturated fat, and total fat and a higher intake of fruit, vegetables, and fiber than their nonvegetarian counterparts.[2]*

Do You Know What to Eat?

Dietitians also support the health aspects of a vegetarian diet. In a position statement published in the *Journal of the American Dietetic Association*, the ADA and Dietitians of Canada stated: "Appropriately planned vegetarian diets are healthful, nutritionally adequate, and provide health benefits in the prevention and treatment of certain diseases."[3]

Why Choose Vegetarianism?

Health concerns are not the only reason people choose to follow vegetarian diets. Being a vegetarian sometimes involves political, religious, or ethical views. For example, since about the 1960s, animal rights groups have been politically active in spreading their message that nonhuman animals have a right to be free from pain and suffering and that slaughtering animals for food is cruel, unhealthy, and immoral. Morally inspired vegetarians are generally antiviolence, and some believe that there is no difference between meat eaters and cannibals—both eat meat derived from animals, they contend. In addition, such ethical vegetarians argue that the earth's productive land could grow much more food for humans per acre if grains, vegetables, and other plant foods were raised for human consumption rather than for animal feed.

Among religious vegetarians are Seventh-Day Adventists, which is a Protestant group that advocates a vegetarian diet as part of its spiritual and health practices. Health emphasis has been part of the church since its beginning in the 1860s. One of its leaders, Mrs. Ellen G. White, believed that any abuse of the body was a violation of God's temple. Long before nutrition became a science, White was advising Adventists to eat a well-balanced diet, to eat natural foods in season, to avoid meat and animal fat, and to reject refined foods, such as white sugar and flour, which she believed even then to be lacking in nutrients.

Today, the Seventh-Day Adventist church includes health and healing practices as a basic part of its teachings. The church operates hospitals, clinics, university medical schools, and centers.

Beyond Vegetables

Newcomers to vegetarian eating are certainly familiar with vegetables, fruits, and nuts, but they may not know about other items that are common in a vegetarian diet. They include:

brewer's yeast—A nutritional yeast not used for baking but a good source of B vitamins and protein that can be added to a variety of foods.

bulgur wheat—A whole grain that is parboiled, dried, then cracked. When soaked it becomes fluffy and can be used in many dishes.

hummus (*shown below*)—A puree of chickpeas and sesame seed paste seasoned with lemon juice and garlic that is used as a spread and dip.

kefir—A cultured milk product that is like liquid yogurt.

millet—A grain that can be used in place of rice and provides protein.

miso—A fermented soybean paste that is a base for soups and a source of protein.

tempeh—A meat substitute made from soybeans.

tofu—A curd made from soybean milk that is curdled in much the same way as cow's milk is curdled for cottage cheese.

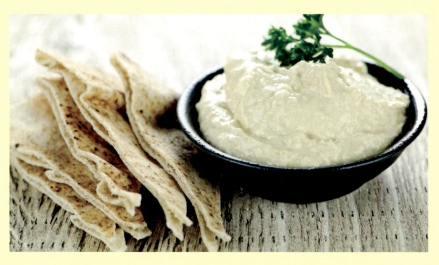

Do You Know What to Eat?

Health food industries are part of the church complex, also. Food companies affiliated with the Adventists process and package goods that contain no meat, animal shortening, refined sugar, or flour.

Several other religious groups in the United States practice vegetarianism. For instance, many Hindus, but not all, avoid meat, which is a practice based on veneration of the life cycle. Most do not eat beef. Thousands of years ago, Hindus in India placed a taboo on killing cows except in times of famine. Since then the cow has been considered sacred in Hinduism.

Other Eastern religions also practice vegetarianism. Jains, followers of an ancient religion that developed along with Hinduism and Buddhism in India, believe that it is wrong to kill any living creature and practice *ahimsa*—a Sanskrit word for nonviolence. Buddhism and Taoism are two more religions that encourage vegetarian eating as a means of respecting nature and living beings.

In recent years, an increasing number of Christians of diverse denominations have chosen vegetarian lifestyles as a component of their religious beliefs. One group that espouses this view is the international Christian Vegetarian Association (CVA), which spreads its message on its Web site and at church conventions. One part of its mission is, "To show the world that plant-based diets represent good, responsible Christian stewardship for all God's Creation." On its Web page, the CVA also states, "We encourage vegetarianism because the diet is ecologically sound, helps alleviate world hunger, and benefits human health."[4]

Recipes for vegetarian dishes are available on the Internet, in hundreds of books about vegetarianism, cookbooks, newspapers, and magazines. Some recipes are based on ethnic cuisine—using flavors from Greece, Italy, Asia, and Latin America. Tabouli, for example, is a popular Mediterranean dish that many vegetarians enjoy. It is made with two cups of bulgur wheat soaked in one cup of warm or boiling water. The wheat is then mixed with chopped scallions, parsley, tomatoes, and a mixture of 1/4 cup lemon juice and 1/2 cup olive oil, garlic salt, and pepper to taste. The tabouli is

What Vegetarians Eat

usually placed in the refrigerator for a few hours to allow the flavors to blend.

Because hamburgers are such popular American fare, a vegetarian substitute can be made with tofu and potatoes. In a blender, grind two small peeled potatoes and 12 ounces of firm tofu with 1/4 cup each of garbanzo beans, whole wheat flour, and chopped walnuts, two small onions, one vegetable bouillon cube, one tablespoon dry yeast, and salt, pepper, garlic powder, and soy sauce to taste. Make patties from the mixture and brown on both sides in a frying pan.

From Traditional Foods to Vegetarian Meals

Is it difficult to make the transition from a meat-based diet to vegetarian eating? That is a question many people ask. The answer is simply no if a person starts with meals that he or she usually eats. For example, refried vegetarian beans can be substituted for the meat in a burrito, and if dairy products are consumed, add cheese. Chili can be made without meat by substituting textured vegetable protein. The other ingredients could include red beans or kidney beans, tomato sauce, onions, green pepper, and other vegetables of one's choice. Chili mac can consist of the chili ingredients plus macaroni and corn.

A pizza made with pita bread, tomato sauce, and vegetables is a good substitute for a meat-covered pizza whether made at home or ordered from a fast food source. Tacos with refried beans and vegetables and stir-fred vegetables with tofu and brown rice are two more simple alternatives. Other alternatives include a vegetable fajita, vegetable stews, and soups made with a vegetarian broth. There are also ready-made items in supermarkets, such as veggie burgers, veggie hot dogs, soy pepperoni, and cheese slices.

Salads, of course, are easily part of a vegetarian diet when they are made without meat or poultry toppings. Cheese and eggs may also be eliminated for some vegetarians. A favorite salad for many vegetarians is made with beans—kidney beans, garbanzo beans,

Do You Know What to Eat?

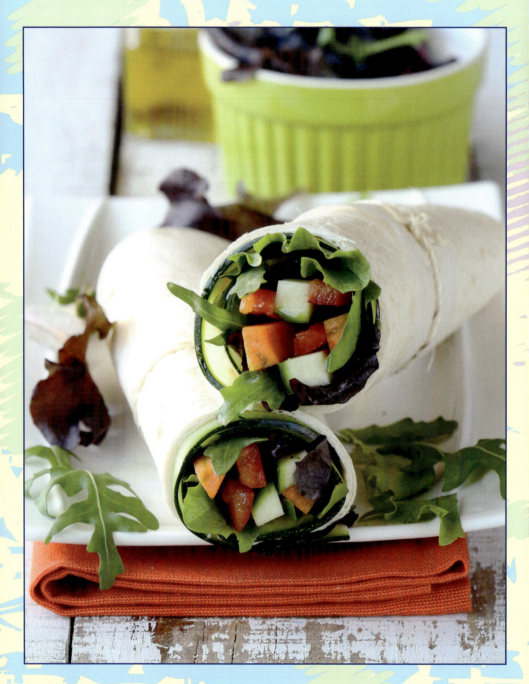

Veggie wraps are a great alternative to a meat and cheese sandwich. Most delis and school cafeterias offer healthy meatless wrap sandwiches for vegetarians.

What Vegetarians Eat

green and wax beans, onions, and a sweetened vinegar dressing. Fruit salad is another popular option.

What about eating at the school cafeteria? In some cases, vegetarian students make and bring their lunches from home. Colleges are more likely to offer vegetarian foods in cafeterias and dorms than are secondary schools. But some middle schools and high schools do offer vegetarian items or have stations for vegetarian foods, such as salads and cheese pizza. The latter can be greasy, unpalatable, and taboo for vegetarians who do not eat dairy products. However, a few schools are starting vegetarian lunch lines that offer much more variety from pasta salad to veggie egg rolls.

Is it possible for a vegetarian to eat out? Many large cities now have vegetarian or vegetarian friendly restaurants, which are listed in the advertisement pages of telephone books or in tour guides. Vegetarian dishes are also available in fast food restaurants ranging from Applebee's to Wendy's. Some menus explain whether meat fats are used in cooking and whether dairy products are contained in baked goods.

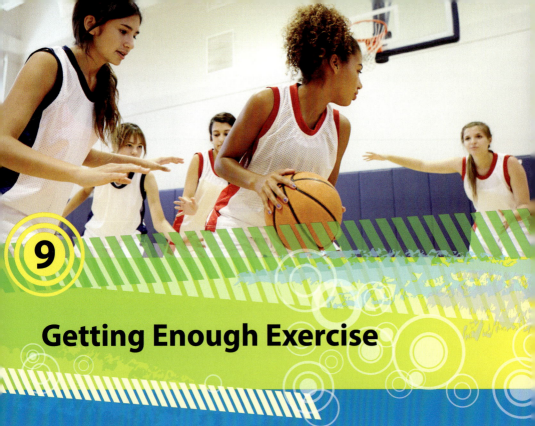

9

Getting Enough Exercise

Advice about eating nutritious food comes from many sources, and it is accompanied by recommendations for physical activity. The USDA's choosemyplate.gov says, "Physical activity and nutrition work together for better health. Being active increases the amount of calories burned. As people age their metabolism slows, so maintaining energy balance requires moving more and eating less." [1]

Many Americans, including students from the elementary grades through high school, are not getting sufficient exercise. The lack of regular physical activity can lead to health risks, such as heart disease and obesity. "If you're not exercising, you're putting yourself at risk for developing a number of serious health conditions. But if you are getting regular physical activity, the opposite is true— you're actually protecting yourself against those diseases and

Getting Enough Exercise

improving your health," writes Diana Rodriguez on livestrong.com. She explains,

> Regular exercise can protect your heart, keep blood pressure and cholesterol levels healthy, maintain a healthy body weight, and protect against diabetes. All of these issues are risk factors for suffering a stroke, so exercise also helps to protect against stroke. Exercise also helps to protect against depression and helps you better manage stress. [2]

In addition, exercise contributes to healthy bones, muscles, and joints.

Physical Activity in Schools

The Health and Human Services Administration (HHSA) reviewed numerous studies regarding the relationship between physical activity and academic performance and issued a report in July 2010 that noted, "There is substantial evidence that physical activity can help improve academic achievement, including grades and standardized test scores." In its review, the HHSA also confirmed:

> When children and adolescents participate in the recommended level of physical activity—at least 60 minutes daily—multiple health benefits accrue. Most youth, however, do not engage in recommended levels of physical activity. Schools provide a unique venue for youth to meet the activity recommendations, as they serve nearly 56 million youth. At the same time, schools face increasing challenges in allocating time for physical education and physical activity during the school day. [3]

In 2013, First Lady Michelle Obama announced a school exercise project called Let's Move and promised "more than $100 million in public and private money to help schools develop physical activity programs for their students," according to *USA TODAY*. She pointed out that schools have a hard time finding time and money "to help our kids be active. . . . But just because it's hard doesn't mean we should stop trying—it means we should try harder." [4]

Do You Know What to Eat?

Physical Education Classes

Periodically, the National Association for Sport and Physical Education (NASPE) and the AHA produce a report titled *Shape of the Nation*. The 2010 report noted:

> Physical education is based on a sequence of learning. These formalized courses are taught by professionals and focus on the skills and knowledge needed to establish and sustain an active lifestyle. Physical education classes focus on physical activity—running, dancing and other movement, but physical education also includes health, nutrition, social responsibility, and the value of fitness throughout one's life. . . .

According to the report, "Only five states in the country—Illinois, Iowa, Massachusetts, New Mexico, and Vermont—require physical education in every grade K-12. New Jersey and Rhode Island require physical education in grades 1-12." However, thirty-two states allow substitutes for physical education, such as marching band and cheerleading.

In its recommendations, NASPE and AHA say:

> School-age youths need at least 60 minutes of moderate-to-vigorous physical activity every day. To achieve that level of activity, NASPE and AHA recommend that schools across the country make physical education the cornerstone of a comprehensive school physical activity program that also includes health education, elementary school recess, after-school physical activity clubs and intramurals, high school interscholastic athletics, walk/bike-to-school programs, and staff wellness programs. It is particularly important that voluntary programs (i.e., after-school physical activity clubs, intramurals) are designed to attract all students, especially those not interested in traditional athletic programs.[5]

Promoting Healthy Eating and Physical Activity

Along with the Let's Move program, other efforts to counteract the health risks associated with inactivity include the CDC's KidsWalk-

Getting Enough Exercise

to-School. It is a community-based program that encourages children to walk or ride a bike short distances to and from school. Several decades ago, the majority of students walked or rode bikes to school, but currently walking and bicycling are dangerous due to heavy vehicle traffic, fear of abductions, and neighborhood crime.

The KidsWalk program encourages civic leaders, parents, school personnel, police, and others to get involved and create safe routes for students. The program's goals include increasing awareness of the health benefits of regular physical activity and improving walkways, crosswalks, and bike paths so that students do not have to be driven or bused to school.

The National Alliance for Nutrition and Activity (NANA) is also a major promoter of physical education in schools. Its members represent more than four hundred organizations concerned about healthy living. One of NANA's primary goals is to promote children's health and well-being. Advocates urge the US Congress and federal agencies to provide adequate funding for programs and environmental changes that help Americans eat better and be more active.

NANA also developed *Model School Wellness Policies on Physical Activity and Nutrition,* which school districts with federally funded meal programs developed and began operating during the 2006–2007 school year. Since then, school districts have adapted the policies to fit their circumstances, but the model basically sets forth goals, such as:

- community involvement in school nutrition and physical activity efforts
- opportunities for all students in grades K–12 to be physically active on a regular basis
- access to a variety of affordable, nutritious, and appealing foods that meet the health and nutrition needs of students
- nutrition education and physical education to foster lifelong healthy habits.[6]

Do You Know What to Eat?

In some states, physical activity is being promoted by nontraditional means, such as exertainment—a term that combines exercise and entertainment that was coined by the audiovisual and video industry. One example is Dance Dance Revolution (DDR), a music-based video game produced by Konami Digital Entertainment, a Japanese company. The game has been available for use in US homes and arcades since 1999. In 2007, West Virginia, a state with a high rate of obesity, introduced the dance program in all of its public schools' physical education classes. DDR has many variations. Players choose a song and operate the game with a dance pad that corresponds with four arrows that point forward, back, left, and right on a screen. Watching the screen, players follow various sequences on the floor mat alone or with a partner. They can also engage in competitions.

In 2013, Konami introduced Dance Dance Revolution Classroom Edition, which was designed specifically for physical education classes. As many as forty-eight students can participate at one time. Each student has a wireless mat that features a smart card reader. While students move to the beat, teachers can see their progress, including steps, body mass index, and calories burned.

Skate In School is another nontraditional program encouraging student physical activity. It was developed by Rollerblade and the National Association of Sports and Physical Education. Schools purchase Rollerblade skates and protective gear (helmets and wrist, elbow, and knee guards) at reduced prices, along with instructions for physical education classes. In 2010, Rollerblade declared on its website that the program was operating in one thousand schools across the country with an estimated three million students involved. [7]

A variety of school clubs are also helping promote physical fitness among youth. There are unicycle clubs, for instance, that engage students in vigorous exercise on the unicycle on school playgrounds, tennis courts, or parking lots. School-sponsored skateboard and surfboard clubs are popular on the West Coast.

Getting Enough Exercise

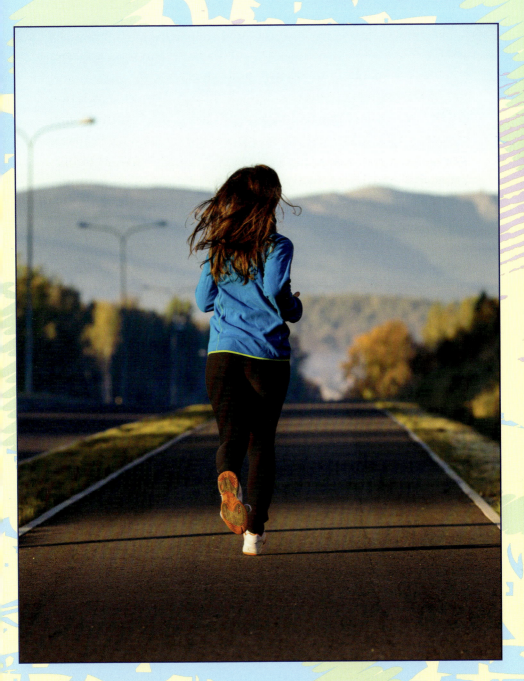

Regular exercise benefits both the body and the mind. Jogging is a healthy activity that can be done almost anywhere and doesn't require any extra equipment.

Do You Know What to Eat?

Obviously there are diverse ways to participate in physical activity. The point is to make it a regular part of one's daily life. The CDC recommends at least sixty minutes per day of moderate to vigorous physical activity for children and youth, although some experts suggest that ninety minutes of daily physical activity would be better. That time could be broken up into shorter periods that add up to an hour or more of individual sports, hiking, biking, swimming, dancing, physical education, gardening, or other physical tasks. It is a matter of using up calories and adding to the health benefits achieved through a nutritious eating plan.

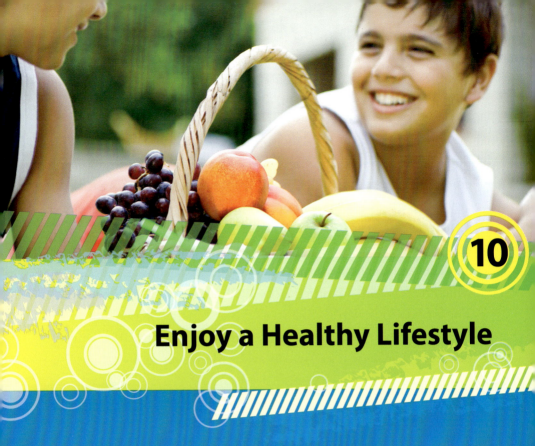

Enjoy a Healthy Lifestyle

Sometimes people think that eating healthy food can be boring. They fear that they won't enjoy their meals or snacks or that they will have to give up foods and beverages they really like. That is not the case, however. In the first place, a healthy diet does not consist of one set of specific foods and beverages. It can be imaginative and varied.

One person who put his imagination to work for healthy eating was Shawn DeMartino of Cape Cod, Massachusetts. Shawn started cooking and experimenting with recipes when he was only eleven years old. At the time, he said he was overweight ("pudgy") and began exercising to slim down. He added healthy food to his regimen by cooking the evening meals for his family. One of his recipes is for a pizza with plenty of vegetables and boneless, skinless chicken breast. He also made tacos with grilled fish—tilapia or mahi mahi—stuffed inside soft corn tortillas. He added avocado salsa and shredded

Do You Know What to Eat?

cabbage. "Through cooking, you learn to eat right," Shawn told a reporter. "And it stays with you for your whole life. If you start cooking as a kid, most times you keep those habits."[1]

In 2010, Shawn explained to the Mark Bavis Leadership Foundation, "[As] I became more aware of the growing national childhood obesity pandemic, I realized my own potential to exact change in the lives of other children experiencing the same difficulties."[2] Shawn has appeared on the *Rachael Ray* cooking show, and through media interviews he has inspired his peers to eat in a healthy manner. He wrote a Cook Booklet with some of his recipes, which he has sent to young people who want help losing weight. The foundation awarded Shawn a scholarship that helped him enter Harvard University in the fall of 2010; he graduated in 2014. During his years at Harvard, he was an avid polo player and captain of a men's team.

Teen Views About Healthy Living

Writing for *Teen Ink,* numerous teenagers have much to say about food, exercise, and healthy lifestyles. Kennard B. of Washington, D.C., is one example. He wrote:

> *Healthy eating is a big part of my life. People that are not eating healthy should. . . because it is worth the rewards at the end. Eating healthy is not something you have to do, but is something you should do. I say this because you will not be judged as much, you can lose weight, and your body will be healthier.* [3]

An anonymous writer in Crested Butte, Colorado, declared: "Eating healthy is important for everyone, especially teens. A healthy diet is the key to being fit." [4]

Alaya of Perrysburg, Ohio, who is another *Teen Ink* contributor, wrote:

> *Being healthy is not just about what you eat, even though that is a big portion. Being healthy is about how you treat your body, meaning what you put into it and the type of things you put your*

body through. Most people think being healthy is an expensive and difficult lifestyle. It is really not much different or much more expensive than the way that most people live now. People are just reluctant to make changes in their lives. So these are merely excuses that hold people back from leading healthy lives.[5]

On New York City's "Teen Speak" website, dozens of contributors express their opinions about physical activity and healthy eating. Here are some examples:

"Being active gives me more energy, not less. When I spend too much time just sitting around, that's when I feel lazy and tired."—Carlos, 16

"I used to run out of breath and look like an idiot compared to other guys. I hated gym class! Then I met this girl and we started playing tennis. Now I try to do some physical activity every day because the feeling at the end is worth it. . . . The best reward is being able to keep up with those guys who once laughed at me."—Erick, 18

"It's not that hard to do an hour of physical activity a day. I just go out and play sports with my friends or with people I meet in the park."—Jessica, 15

Healthy food and beverages are also topics that prompt comments. Fifteen-year-old Elizabeth notes: "Most parents, like mine, fill up your plate with ridiculous amounts of food and don't let you get up from the table until it's all gone. Little by little, you get used to eating large portions. But more food isn't necessarily better. Smaller portions can be just as nutritious."

"I always used to skip the food at school and go home and eat junk food. I gained 20 pounds in 3 months. You don't want to make the same mistake I did," fifteen-year-old Dede advises.

Eighteen-year-old David says: "Most people grab a soda instead of water when they are thirsty. With so many soda ads, it makes

Do You Know What to Eat?

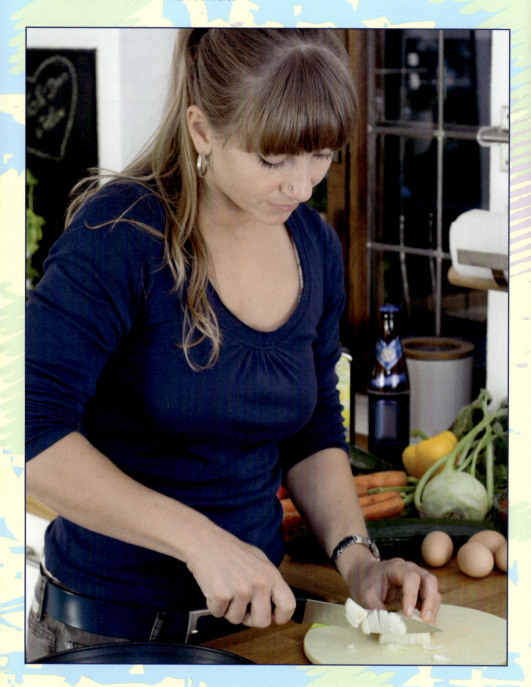

Studies show that cooking together as a family can help promote healthy eating behaviors early on. Home-cooked meals are often healthier than store-bought meals.

Enjoy a Healthy Lifestyle

sense that we automatically pick soda over water even though water is a better choice."

Chanely, age thirteen, agrees: "I always ordered a soda with everything I ate. Recently, however, I began breaking out horribly. I was willing to try anything to clear my skin. To my surprise, after I quit soda and started drinking water, my pimples almost disappeared. I feel better than ever." [6]

Eating Routines

Most teens who want to develop healthy eating routines may begin by following the advice of numerous health experts—start the morning by eating breakfast. Studies show that those who eat breakfast have healthier body weights and better academic success than non-breakfast eaters. Eating breakfast also prevents the run-down feeling, or the lack of energy that can occur midmorning because the body has insufficient fuel. By lunchtime, a person may be not only hungry but also irritable and primed to eat nonnutritious, calorie-laden foods.

What is a healthy breakfast? One that contains protein, such as eggs, low-fat meat, or beans, and fiber, such as whole grain cereal and fruit. Another example is a vegetable omelet with a bran muffin and orange juice. A nutritious breakfast is even possible while eating on the go. One take-along is a whole wheat pita stuffed with sliced hard-boiled eggs. Another is a bagel with peanut butter and some apple slices.

Healthy eating customs also include meals with the family—particularly dinner or supper. That may be difficult to establish, especially when some family members have after-school activities while others have evening work schedules or volunteer commitments. But a family meal does not have to be in the evening. It can occur whenever everyone can be together—breakfast, lunch, dinner, or even a regular snack time.

The importance of the eating together as a family has been underscored by a number of studies. One of them was conducted by

Do You Know What to Eat?

Project EAT (Educate, Act, Thrive). According to the US National Library of Medicine's PubMed 2010 article:

> Many adolescents and parents view family meals in a positive light, but there is great diversity in the context and frequency of family meal patterns in the homes of adolescents. . . . Findings from Project EAT, in conjunction with other research studies on family meals, suggest the importance of working with families to increase the frequency and improve the quality of family meals. Further research is needed in order to elucidate the pathways that underpin the relationships between family meals and health outcomes. [7]

What about eating fast food at the family dinner table? Some researchers say that when families eat fast food at mealtimes, the fewer fruits and vegetables they consume. They are also likely to have salty snacks and sugary soft drinks available. But no one suggests eliminating fast food altogether. Instead, it is a matter of limiting fast foods and adding more fruits, vegetables, whole grains, and low-fat milk.

Suggestions for Enjoyable Eating

It has been said and written so often that it is like a mantra: Healthy eating means consuming fruits and vegetables, whole grains, unsaturated fats, and low-calorie foods and beverages. Are there simple ways to obtain these foods and still have an enjoyable eating experience?

Snacks made at home are a good way to start. Some examples include an apple with peanut butter, celery topped with peanut butter and raisins, trail mix, baby carrots and cherry tomatoes with a low-fat dip, or whole grain crackers and string cheese.

Adding fruits and vegetables to one's diet can be as simple as mixing a whole grain cereal with dried or fresh fruit or spreading a mashed banana or berries on whole wheat toast. You can also eat fruit for dessert, make a full meal of vegetable soup, drink a fruit

Enjoy a Healthy Lifestyle

smoothie or veggie quencher, or eat casseroles with more vegetables than meat or poultry.

It is a little more difficult to choose a healthy meal when you are eating out. But a few dos and don'ts may help:

- Do keep portions small.
- Do not supersize—try cutting a sandwich in half, for example.
- Do eat a lot of greens, especially salads with low-fat dressing.
- Do not load up salads or other foods with lots of cheese, croutons, or other extras.
- Do eat grilled meats, poultry, and fish rather than fried.
- Do not habitually opt for fried, deep-fried, and breaded foods.
- Do drink low-calorie and low- or no-sugar beverages.
- Do not give up ALL foods that happen to be high in calories and saturated fat, but eat them sparingly.

Finally, here is good advice from an anonymous teenager who explained in *Teen Ink* why healthy eating is so important:

> *It can prevent and control health problems. It has shown to help and prevent heart disease, high blood pressure, Type 2 diabetes, and even some cancers. It is not the same as going on a diet. Diets are temporary and make you eat less food rather than the right food. Dieting can cause your body to not get the nutrients it needs, while eating healthy boosts and balances the amount of nutrients in your body. But how do you start your healthy diet? You have to aim for balance in the different food groups. Make sure you look for a variety, it helps you get the nutrition you need. Overall, you need to pay attention to what you eat. You need to stay balanced to make sure you have enough vitamin and minerals. It also improves your mood, helps you handle stress, and gives you more energy.* [8]

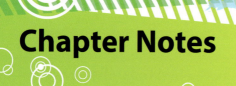

Chapter Notes

Chapter 1: Eating While Socializing

1. Centers for Disease Control and Prevention, "Childhood Obesity Facts," <http://www.cdc.gov/obesity/data/childhood.html> (November 26, 2014).
2. New York City Department of Health and Mental Hygiene, *Teen Speak...about Getting Fit,* p. 6, <http://www.nyc.gov/html/doh/downloads/pdf/cdp/cdp_teensspeakfit.pdf> (November 26, 2014).

Chapter 2: What's in A Name?

1. Elaine Magee, MPH, RD, "Junk-Food Facts," WebMD, n.d., <webmd.com/diet/features/junk-food-facts> (November 27, 2014).
2. National Heart, Lung, and Blood Institute, "Making the Best Choice: How To Choose a Healthier Fast Food Meal," n.d., <http://www.nhlbi.nih.gov/files/docs/resources/heart/filipino-health-manual/appendix/best.pdf> (November 27, 2014).
3. Astrid, "The Importance of Healthy Eating," teenspeak.org, November 3, 2014, <http://teenspeak.org/2014/11/03/the-importance-of-healthy-eating/> (November 27, 2014).
4. US Food and Drug Administration, "FDA Finalizes Menu and Vending Machine Calorie Labeling Rules," news release, November 25, 2014, <http://www.foodpolitics.com/wp-content/uploads/Embargoed-FDA-News-Release.pdf> (November 27, 2014).
5. <http://ghr.nlm.nih.gov/handbook/howgeneswork/protein> (November 27, 2014).
6. Walter Willet, "The Scientific Case for Banning Trans Fats,"

scientificamerican.com, March 1, 2014, <http://www.scientificamerican.com/article/scientific-case-for-banning-trans-fats/> (November 28, 2014).

7. American Heart Association, "Trans Fat," updated August 5, 2014, <http://www.heart.org/HEARTORG/GettingHealthy/NutritionCenter/HealthyEating/Trans-Fats_UCM_301120_Article.jsp> (November 28, 2014).

8. Dr. Frank Sacks, "Ask the Expert: Omega-3 Fatty Acids," hsph.harvard.edu, n.d., <http://www.hsph.harvard.edu/nutritionsource/omega-3/> (November 28, 2014).

9. <http://www.heart.org/HEARTORG/GettingHealthy/NutritionCenter/HealthyDietGoals/Fish-and-Omega-3-Fatty-Acids_UCM_303248_Article.jsp> (November 28, 2014).

Chapter 3: Our Eating Practices

1. Gillian Crowther, *Eating Culture: An Anthropological Guide to Food* (Toronto, Ontario, Canada: University of Toronto Press, 2013), paperback edition, p. 152.

2. Lifespan. "Family, Friends, Social Ties Influence Weight Status In Young Adults." *ScienceDaily*, January 13, 2011, <www.sciencedaily.com/releases/2011/01/110111133023.htm> (November 28, 2014).

3. David Cameron, "Obesity Spreads through Social Networks," Harvard Medical School Office of Public Affairs, July 26, 2007, <http://web.med.harvard.edu/sites/RELEASES/html/July07Christakis.html> (October 5, 2007).

4. Gina Kolata, "Find Yourself Packing It On? Blame Friends," *New York Times*, July 26, 2007, <http://www.nytimes.com/2007/07/26/health/26fat.html?ex=1186286400&en=518926e6eb95cafa&ei=5070> (October 5, 2007).

Do You Know What to Eat?

5. Kadesha McCastle, "Unhealthy Eating Habits," _Youth Radio Atlanta_, October 7, 2006, <http://www.youthradio.org/health/wabe061007_badfoods.shtml> (October 5, 2007).

6. Denae Bybee, "Young Girl Fights Obesity and Tells of Her Struggles," _BYU (Brigham Young University) NewsNet_, August 4, 2007, <http://newsnet.byu.edu/story.cfm/65002> (October 5, 2007).

7. Harvard School of Public Health, news release, "Skipping Breakfast May Increase Coronary Heart Disease Risk," hsph.harvard.edu, July 23, 2013, <http://www.hsph.harvard.edu/news/features/skipping-breakfast-may-increase-coronary-heart-disease-risk/> (December 1, 2013).

8. Supplemental Assistance Nutrition Program <http://www.fns.usda.gov/snap/eligibility> (December 1, 2014).

Chapter 4: Poor Eating Habits Impair Health

1. Rudd Center for Food Policy and Obesity, "Food Marketing to Youth," 2013, <http://www.yaleruddcenter.org/what_we_do.aspx?id=4> (December 3, 2014).

2. Marlene B. Schwartz and Amy Ustjanauskas, "Food Marketing to Youth: Current Threats and Opportunities," _Childhood Obesity_, April 2012, p. 86-87, <http://www.yaleruddcenter.org/resources/upload/docs/what/advertising/FoodMarketingYouthThreatsOpportunities_CO_4.12.pdf> (December 3, 2014).

3. Elizabeth B. Rappaport MD, Constantine Daskalakis ScD and Jocelyn Andrel MSPH, "Obesity and Other Predictors of Absenteeism in Philadelphia School Children," _Journal of School Health_, Volume 81, Issue 6, pages 341–344, June 2011.

Chapter Notes

4. <http://www.ncbi.nlm.nih.gov/pubmed/21592129> (December 5, 2014).

5. See <http://www.nature.com/ijo/journal/v36/n4/abs/ijo201215a.html> (December 5, 2014).

6. Centers for Disease Control and Prevention, "Childhood Obesity Facts," cdc.gov, page last reviewed August 13, 2014, <http://www.cdc.gov/healthyyouth/obesity/facts.htm> (December 5, 2014).

7. American Diabetes Association, "Statistics About Diabetes," diabetes.org, June 2014, <http://www.diabetes.org/diabetes-basics/statistics/> (December 5, 2014).

8. <http://www.diabetes.org/diabetes-basics/myths/> (December 5, 2014).

9. Valerie Liles, "The Effects of Nutrition on the Respiratory System," lifestrong.com, February 9, 2014, <http://www.livestrong.com/article/391677-the-effects-of-nutrition-on-the-respiratory-system/> (December 5, 2014).

Chapter 5: Dangerous Eating Behaviors

1. The Eating Disorder Foundation, "About Eating Disorders," 2013, <eatingdisorderfoundation.org/EatingDisorders.htm> (December 6, 2014).

2. Ron Saxen, *The Good Eater: The True Story of One Man's Struggle with Binge Eating Disorder* (Oakland, Calif.: New Harbinger Publications, 2007), p. 3.

3. University of Maryland Medical Center, "Eating Disorders," last updated June 24, 2013, <http://umm.edu/health/medical/reports/articles/eating-disorders> (December 6, 2014).

4. <http://www.ncsl.org/documents/statefed/health/MHParity-FRule_mwedits.pdf> (December 6, 2014).

5. Anorexia Nervosa and Related Eating Disorders, "What Causes

Do You Know What to Eat?

Eating Disorders?" anred.com, 2011, <http://www.anred.com/causes.html> (December 6, 2014).

6. Loren Thomas, "Surviving and Eating Disorder: Two Teens Speak Out," newsplex.com, February 11, 2014, <http://www.newsplex.com/home/headlines/Surviving-and-Eating-Disorder-Two-Teens-Speak-Out-244986181.html> (December 6, 2014).

7. Anorexia Nervosa and Related Eating Disorders, Inc., "Statistics: How Many People Have Eating Disorders?" 2011, <http://www.anred.com/stats.html> (December 7, 2014).

Chapter 6: Do You Eat for Good Health?

1. *Dietary Guidelines for Americans, 2010*, Chapter 5, health.gov, December 2010, <http://www.health.gov/dietaryguidelines/dga2010/DietaryGuidelines2010.pdf> (December 7, 2014).

2. "What's On Your Plate?" choosemyplate.gov, August 2011, <http://www.choosemyplate.gov/downloads/mini_poster_English_final.pdf> (December 7, 2014).

3. Melanie A. Guzman, "Harvard School of Public Health Creates Nutrition Guide," thecrimson.com, September 15, 2011, <http://www.thecrimson.com/article/2011/9/15/healthy-plate-eating-food/> (December 15, 2014).

4. Harvard School of Public Health, "New US Dietary Guidelines: Progress, Not Perfection," <http://www.hsph.harvard.edu/nutritionsource/dietary-guidelines-2010/> (December 7, 2014).

5. United States Department of Agriculture, "Healthier School Day," fns.usda.gov, September 29, 2014, <http://www.fns.usda.gov/healthierschoolday/tools-schools-focusing-smart-snacks> (December 7, 2014).

6. <http://www.fns.usda.gov/sites/default/files/NSLPFactSheet.pdf> (December 8, 2014).

Chapter Notes

7. University of Connecticut, "Local Routes," <http://dining.uconn.edu/local-routes/> (December 8, 2014).

8. "Congressional Food Stamp Challenge," June 2007, <http://foodstampchallenge.typepad.com/> (December 9, 2014).

9. Representative Barbara Lee, "Join Members of Congress, Take the #SNAPChallenge," huffingtonpost.com, June 12, 2013 updates August 13, 2013, <http://www.huffingtonpost.com/rep-barbara-lee/join-members-of-congress_b_3428820.html> (December 8, 2014).

Chapter 7: Dieting Dos and Don'ts

1. Patricia van den Berg, Dianne Neumark-Sztainer, Peter J. Hannan, and Jess Haines, "Is Dieting Advice From Magazines Helpful or Harmful? Five-Year Associations With Weight-Control Behaviors and Psychological Outcomes in Adolescents," *Pediatrics Official Journal of the American Academy of Pediatrics*, Abstract, January 1, 2007, p. e30, <http://pediatrics.aappublications.org/cgi/content/abstract/119/1/e30> (December 9, 2014).

2. Katherine Zeratsky, Mayo Clinic Staff, "Do Detox Diets Offer Any Health Benefits?" April 21, 2012, <http://www.mayoclinic.com/health/detox-diets/AN01334> (December 10, 2014).

3. American Heart Association, "Quick-Weight-Loss or Fad Diets," March 18, 2014, <http://www.heart.org/HEARTORG/GettingHealthy/NutritionCenter/Quick-Weight-Loss-or-Fad-Diets_UCM_305970_Article.jsp> (December 10, 2014).

4. Ibid.

5. Natalie Smith, "Diet Pills and Teenagers," livestrong.com, July 10, 2011, <http://www.livestrong.com/article/489043-diet-pills-teenagers/> (December 10, 2014).

6. Mayo Clinic Health Staff, "Over-the-counter weight-loss pills: Do

Do You Know What to Eat?

they work?" February 11, 2012, <http://www.mayoclinic.com/ health/ weight-loss/HQ01160> (December 10, 2014).

7. US Food and Drug Administration, "Dietary Supplements," updated November 13, 2014, <http://www.fda.gov/Food/ DietarySupplements/> (December 10, 2014).

8. Consumer Reports, "Legal Ephedra?" ConsumerReports.org, March 2010, <http://www.consumerreports.org/cro/magazine-archive/2010/march/health/ephedra/overview/ephedra-ov.htm> (December 10, 2014).

9. Benjamin Plackett, "Ads for Over The Counter Drugs Are Worse Than Those That Require A Prescription," insidescience.org, September 26, 2013, <http://www.insidescience.org/content/ study-finds-most-drug-commercials-misleading/1418> (December 10, 2014).

10. <http://www.cdc.gov/pcd/issues/2013/12_0224.htm> (December 10, 2014).

11. Public Citizen, "New York City's Fast-Food Calorie Labeling Rule Should Be Upheld, Groups Urge Federal Court," Press Release, July 16, 2007, <http://www.citizen.org/pressroom/release.cfm?ID= 2476> (December 10, 2014).

12. US Department of Health and Human Services, Weight-control Information Network (WIN), "Just Enough for You—About Food Portions," June 2009, updated March 2012, <http://win.niddk.nih. gov/publications/just_enough.htm> (December 10, 2014).

Chapter 8: What Vegetarians Eat

1. American Heart Association, "Vegetarian Diets," n.d., <http:// www. americanheart.org/presenter.jhtml?identifier=4777> (December 11, 2014).

2. Laurie Dunham and Linda M. Kollar, "Vegetarian Eating for

Chapter Notes

Children and Adolescents," Abstract and Introduction, *Journal of Pediatric Health Care, Medscape,* January 23, 2006, <http:// www.medscape.com/viewarticle/521903> (December 11, 2014).

3. "Position of the American Dietetic Association and Dieticians of Canada: Vegetarian Diets," *Journal of the American Dietetic Association,* June 2003, p. 748.

4. "Our Mission," Christian Vegetarian Association, 2005, <http:// www.all-creatures.org/cva/mission.htm> (December 11, 2014).

Chapter 9: Getting Enough Exercise

1. US Department of Agriculture, "Why Is Physical Activity Important?" choosemyplate.gov, <http://www.choosemyplate.gov/physical-activity/why.html> (December 11, 2014).

2. Diana Rodriguez, "Health Problems and Lack of Exercise," livestrong.com, August 16, 2013, <http://www.livestrong.com/article/412043-health-problems-and-lack-of-exercise/> (December 11, 2014).

3. <http://www.cdc.gov/healthyYouth/health_and_academics/pdf/pa-pe_paper.pdf> (December 11, 2014).

4. David Jackson, "Michelle Obama Launches School Exercise Program," usatoday.com, February 28, 2013, <ww.usatoday.com/story/theoval/2013/02/28/michelle-obama-lets-move-active-schools/1954137/> (December 11, 2014).

5. See *Shape of the Nation Report 2010,* p. 3, 7, 9, <http://www.heart.org/idc/groups/heart-public/@wcm/@adv/documents/downloadable/ucm_308261.pdf> (December 11, 2014).

6. Model School Wellness Policies, n.d., <http://www.schoolwellnesspolicies.org/WellnessPolicies.html> (December 12, 2014).

7. Rollerblade Skate in School, March 1, 2010, <http://www.

101

Do You Know What to Eat?

rollerblade.com/usa/the-rollerblade-experience/kids/rollerblade-skate-in-school/> (December 12, 2014).

Chapter 10: Enjoy a Healthy Lifestyle

1. Gwenn Friss, "Healthy Eating on Cape Teen's Menu," *Cape Cod Times*, September 5, 2007, <http://www.capecodonline.com/apps/pbcs.dll/article?AID=/20070905/LIFE/709050301> (May 9, 2008).

2. "2010 Recipient," <http://www.markbavisleadershipfoundation.org/?p=141> (December 12, 2014).

3. Kennard B. "Eating Healthy," teenink.com, n.d., <http://www.teenink.com/hot_topics/health/article/607061/Eating-Healthy/> (December 13, 2014).

4. Anonymous, "The Importance of Eating Healthy," teenink.com, n.d., <http://www.teenink.com/opinion/all/article/586940/The-Importance-Of-Eating-Healthy/> (December 13, 2014).

5. Alaya, "Healthy Living," teenink.com, n.d., <http://www.teenink.com/hot_topics/health/article/587132/Healthy-Living/> (December 13, 2014).

6. New York City Department of Health and Mental Hygiene, "Teen Speak . . . About Getting Fit," p. 3-10 nyc.gov, n.d., <http://www.nyc.gov/html/doh/downloads/pdf/cdp/cdp_teensspeakfit.pdf> (December 13, 2014).

7. D. Neumark-Sztainer, et. al, National Library of Medicine, PubMed, "Family Meals And Adolescents: What Have We Learned From Project EAT (Eating Among Teens)," July 2010, <http://www.ncbi.nlm.nih.gov/pubmed/20144257> (December 14, 2014).

8. Anonymous, "The Importance of Eating Healthy," teenink.com, n.d., <http://www.teenink.com/opinion/all/article/586940/The-Importance-Of-Eating-Healthy/> (December 13, 2014).

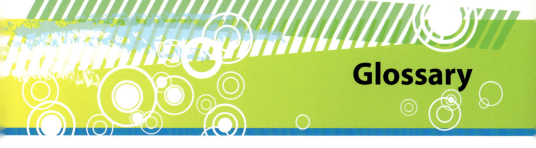

Glossary

amino acids—Strings of molecules that form proteins.

anorexia nervosa—An eating disorder in which a person does not stay at the minimum body weight considered normal for his or her age and height.

binge eating—An eating disorder in which a person has recurrent episodes of significant overeating without purging.

body mass index (BMI)—The most commonly used method of calculating underweight and overweight; the ratio of the weight of the body to the square of its height.

brewer's yeast—A nutritional yeast that is a good source of B vitamins.

bulimia nervosa—An eating disorder in which a person has recurrent episodes of significant overeating followed by purging.

calorie—An energy-producing value in food.

carbohydrates—Nutrients made up of carbon, oxygen, and hydrogen that combine to form sugar molecules that provide most of the energy our bodies need.

cholesterol—A soft waxy substance produced by the body and obtained from food that combines with protein and fatty acids to form LDL (bad cholesterol) and HDL (good cholesterol).

detox diets—Diets that combine fasting with an extremely limited list of foods for a period in order to rid the body of toxins.

diabetes—A disease in which the body does not produce insulin (Type 1) or does not use insulin properly (Type 2).

Do You Know What to Eat?

diabulimia—An eating disorder among Type 1 diabetics who try to lose weight by not taking their insulin.

eating disorder (ED)—A psychological condition that includes a distorted view of self and extreme disturbances in eating behavior.

ephedra (ma huang)—A chemical used in some weight-loss aids, banned in the United States, that can cause serious health complications.

fats—Nutrients made up of fatty acids.

kefir—A cultured milk product similar to liquid yogurt.

lacto-ovo vegetarian—A person who eats no meat or fish but does eat eggs and dairy products.

miso—A fermented soybean paste.

morbid obesity—A medical condition in which a person is a hundred pounds or more over a healthy body weight.

obesity—A condition in which a person has an abnormally high proportion of body fat.

proteins—Nutrients that build and repair body tissues and form antibodies to fight infections. Proteins are made from strings of molecules called amino acids.

purging—Ridding the body of food through such methods as vomiting or laxative abuse.

tempeh—A meat substitute made from soybeans.

tofu—A curd made from soybean milk.

trans fat—A type of fat that occurs naturally in small amounts in food and is also formed when hydrogen is added to vegetable oil to make solid fat.

vegan—A person who eats no animal products.

vegetarian—A person who does not eat meat, fish, fowl, or products made with these foods.

For More Information

Academy of Nutrition and Dietetics

120 South Riverside Plaza, Suite 2000

Chicago, Illinois 60606

(800) 877-1600

eatright.org

American Diabetes Association

1701 North Beauregard Street

Alexandria, VA 22311

(800) 342–2383

diabetes.org

American Heart Association

7272 Greenville Avenue

Dallas, TX 75231

(800) 242–8721

heart.org

American Obesity Treatment Association

117 Anderson Court Suite 1

Dothan, Alabama 36303

(334) 403-4057

americanobesity.org

Centers for Disease Control and Prevention

1600 Clifton Road

Atlanta, GA 30333

(800) 232–4636

cdc.gov

Do You Know What to Eat?

Harvard School of Public Health
677 Huntington Avenue
Boston, MA 02115
(617) 495-1000
hsph.harvard.edu

National Association of Anorexia Nervosa and Associated Disorders
750 E Diehl Road #127
Naperville, IL 60563
(630) 577-1333
anad.org

National Eating Disorders Association
165 West 46th Street Suite 402
New York, NY 10036
(212) 575-6200
nationaleatingdisorders.org

Public Citizen
1600 20th Street NW
Washington, D.C. 20009
(202) 588-1000
citizen.org

US Department of Agriculture
1400 Independence Ave., S.W.
Washington, D.C.
(202) 720-2791
usda.gov

US Department of Health and Human Services
200 Independence Ave., SW
Washington, DC 20201
(877) 696–6775
hhs.gov

For More Information

US Food and Drug Administration

10903 New Hampshire Avenue
Silver Spring, MD 20993
(888) 463-6332
fda.gov

US National Library of Medicine Medline Plus

8600 Rockville Pike
Bethesda, MD 20894
nlm.nih.gov/medlineplus

Web Sites

American Heart Association for Kids

heart.org/HEARTORG/GettingHealthy/HealthierKids/
Healthier-Kids_UCM_304156_SubHomePage.jsp

Choose My Plate

choosemyplate.gov

Let's Move

letsmove.gov

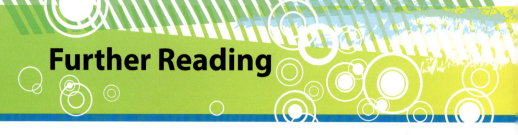

Further Reading

Greene, Jessica. *Eating Disorders: The Ultimate Teen Guide* (It Happened to Me series). Lanham, Md.: Rowman & Littlefield Publishers, 2014

Junger, Alejandro. *Clean Eats: Over 200 Delicious Recipes to Reset Your Body's Natural Balance and Discover What It Means to Be Truly Healthy*. New York, N.Y.: HarperCollins, 2014.

Medford, Christopher G. *Overcoming Binge Eating, Second Edition: The Proven Program to Learn Why You Binge and How You Can Stop*. New York, N.Y.: Guilford Press, 2013.

Sanfilippo, Diane. *Practical Paleo: A Customized Approach to Health and a Whole-Foods Lifestyle*. Riverside, N.J.: Victor Belt Publishing/Simon & Schuster, 2012.

Taubes, Gary. *Why We Get Fat: and What to Do About It*. New York, N.Y.: Anchor Books/Random House, 2011.

Wright, Jonathan and Linda Johnson Larsen. *Eating Clean for Dummies*. Hoboken, N.J.: John Wiley & Sons, 2011.

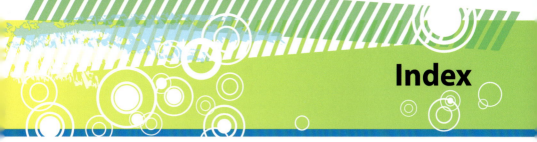

Index

A
absenteeism, 37
American Diabetes Association (ADA), 38-39, 74
American Heart Association (AHA), 21-22, 33, 58, 64-65, 73, 82
amino acids, 16
anorexia, 42, 44-47, 49-50
Anorexia Nervosa and Related Eating Disorders, Inc. (ANRED), 45, 49-50

B
Big Mac, 43
binge eating, 42-43, 46-47, 49-50
blood sugar, 17, 32
body image, 62
body mass index (BMI), 9, 67, 84
breakfast, 12, 23, 27, 31-33, 36, 52, 55, 58, 60, 70, 91
Brownell, Kelly, 29
Buddhism, 76
bulimia, 42-44, 47, 49-50
Burger King, 61

C
calories, 13-15, 19, 30-31, 34, 47, 55-58, 61, 64-65, 68, 70, 73, 80, 84, 86, 91-93

cancer, 11, 22, 37, 53, 64, 73, 93
carbohydrates (carbs), 16-17, 39-40, 55, 63
Cartoon Network, 61
Center for Science in the Public Interest (CSPI), 70
cholesterol, 17, 19, 21, 33, 36, 55, 57-58, 74, 81
Christian Vegetarian Association (CVA), 76
Congressional Food Stamp Challenge, 58

D
daily diet, 13, 19, 25, 62
Dance Dance Revolution (DDR), 84
diabetes, 11, 21, 33, 36-39, 50, 53, 60, 73, 81, 93
diabulimia, 46
dietary guidelines, 19, 51, 55
dietary plan, 34
dietitians, 26, 30, 51, 58, 65, 74
diet pills, 62, 65, 67-68
Disney, 61
Dunkin' Donuts, 21

E
electrolytes, 24, 49
exercise, 13, 30, 33, 39, 40, 46, 50, 60, 80, 81, 84, 88

109

Do You Know What to Eat?

F

family, 7, 27-28, 33-34, 58, 65, 87, 91-92

fast food, 8, 11, 13, 14, 15, 29, 31, 34, 36, 68, 70, 79, 92

fats

    monounsaturated, 20, 57

    polyunsaturated, 20, 21, 57

    saturated, 19, 21, 39-40, 57, 58, 63, 74, 93

    trans, 20-21, 39, 52, 55, 57

fish, 16-17, 20, 22-24, 34, 52-53, 63, 72, 87, 93

food marketing, 61

fried (foods), 13, 21, 54, 93

G

glucose, 17, 36, 38-39

H

Harvard Healthy Eating Plate, 52

Harvard Medical School, 28-29

Harvard School of Public Health, 19, 21-22, 33, 52

heart disease, 11, 16, 19-22, 37, 39-40, 50, 53, 63, 73, 80, 93

I

insulin, 38

J

Johns Hopkins University, 55

junk food, 11, 13-14, 26, 30-31, 33-35, 54, 89

K

Kentucky Fried Chicken (KFC), 15, 21

L

lanugo, 47

M

Mayo Clinic, 26, 64, 67

McDonald's, 14-15, 21, 36, 61

meat, 14, 16-17, 20, 23-24, 34, 52-53, 56, 63, 71-72, 74, 76-77, 79, 91-93

minerals, 11, 16, 22, 24, 49, 57, 93

MyPlate, 26, 51-52, 81

MyPyramid, 26

N

National Association of Sports and Physical Education (NASPE), 82, 84

National Heart, Lung, and Blood Institute (NHLBI), 14

National Institutes of Health (NIH), 26

National School Lunch Program, 54

New York Times, 29

Nutritional Labeling and Education Act, 57

nutrition facts label, 19, 56-57

nutritionist, 14, 26, 47, 51, 65-66

O

obesity, 8-9, 11, 28-29, 32-37,

39, 43, 46, 50, 63, 70, 73, 80, 84, 88
omega-3 (fatty acids), 21, 22
overweight, 8-9, 28, 34, 36-38, 40, 43, 87

P

Patient Protection and Affordable Care Act, 15
physical education, 81-84, 86
pizza, 8, 12, 14, 28, 54, 77, 79, 87
portions, 9, 13, 29, 31, 33-34, 39, 70, 71, 88-89, 93
poultry, 16, 23, 52-53, 71-72, 79, 92-93
Project EAT, 91-92
protein, 11, 16-17, 40, 52-53, 57, 63, 73, 77, 91
Public Citizen, 70
purging, 43, 45, 47, 49-50

S

serving size, 19, 22, 31, 54, 56-58, 70
Seventh-Day Adventists, 74, 76
Shape of the Nation, 82
Skate in School,
Smart Snacks in Schools, 54
snacks, 7, 13, 21, 26, 31, 33, 39, 40-41, 52, 54, 61, 63, 87, 91-92
socializing, 8
soda, 26, 54, 89, 91
sodium (salt), 13, 39, 49, 54-55, 57-58, 60, 63, 77, 92
sports, 7, 82, 84, 86, 89
Starbucks, 21

stroke, 11, 22, 37, 39, 50, 81
Subway, 15
supersize, 29, 93
SuperTracker, The, 52
Supplemental Nutrition Assistance Program (SNAP), 34, 58

T

Taco Bell, 15

U

United States Centers For Disease Control (CDC), 9, 36, 68, 82, 86
United States Department of Agriculture (USDA), 26, 34, 51-52, 54, 80
United States Department of Health and Human Services (DHHS), 15, 51, 81
United States Food and Drug Administration (FDA), 15, 21, 67

V

vegan, 55, 72-73
vegetarian, 12, 55, 72-74, 76-77, 79
veggie burgers, 79
vitamins, 11, 16-17, 22-24, 33, 57, 73, 93

W

water, 16, 25-26, 36, 50, 52, 54, 60, 64, 77, 89, 91
WebMD, 14, 26

Do You Know What to Eat?

Weight-control Information
 Network (WIN), 62, 70
weight-loss diets
 Atkins, 63-64
 Cabbage Soup, 63
 Grapefruit, 63
 Jenny Craig, 65
 South Beach, 63
 Weight Watchers, 65
 Zone, 63
Wendy's, 14-15, 79
whole grains, 12, 14, 23-24, 39,
 52, 54-56, 73, 77, 91-92
Willet, Walter, 21